Time Well Spent
with Epilepsy

Stephen Timewell

ISBN 978-1-964462-80-6 (Paperback)
ISBN 978-1-964462-81-3 (Ebook)

Inquiries and Book Orders should be addressed to:

Leavitt Peak Press
17901 Pioneer Blvd Ste L #298, Artesia, California 90701
Phone #: 2092191548

Other books from Stephen Timewell

Time Well Spent (Published 2010)

A Decade Well Spent (2004 - 2014) (Published 2016)

CONTENTS

INTRODUCTION

What is the purpose of Time Well Spent with Epilepsy? Writing about epilepsy is never easy. What am I trying to achieve in this complex, misunderstood world of medical conundrums, prejudices and extreme diversity? Dictionaries describe epilepsy as 'a neurological disorder marked by sudden recurrent episodes of sensory disturbance, loss of consciousness, or convulsions, associated with abnormal electrical activity in the brain.'

But epilepsy is much more than that and can have a huge impact not only on the direct sufferers but also in the families of those with the diagnosis. Epilepsy is a variable condition that affects different people in different ways and with over 40 different types of seizure, there is extreme diversity and range in the condition.

What seizures look like can vary enormously. Someone may go 'blank' for a couple of seconds, they may wander around and be quite confused, or they may fall to the ground and shake (convulse). Not all seizures involve convulsions and the reasons behind these episodes can be many and varied. This just adds to the complexity surrounding the condition and the difficulty in understanding an individual's situation and what can be done about it.

So why try and write about it? I am not a doctor or a clinician, I am just an ordinary person who has had and lived with epilepsy for over 60 years. And that is the point. This unique, complex condition is not easily understandable by sufferers or their families and over the years many myths, misunderstandings, stigmas and prejudices have emerged which have made the situation even worse.

The range and diversity of the condition has not only made it difficult to describe by practitioners but the emerging myths and misunderstandings have made it even more difficult for the sufferers and their families to deal with it and cope.

So personal accounts of dealing with it and coping take on added significance and meaning. This book is not a solution or cure for those affected by epilepsy but a collection of stories and anecdotes by a person who has been seriously affected by the condition and has been fortunate enough to not let it hinder his progress and development.

I am not a star. But having been told as a young teenager that I would not be able to finish school and never be able to go to university I managed to prove the doctors wrong and finish school and achieve an undergraduate degree in economics in Melbourne and a Masters in Islamic History & Arabic in Chicago as well as a successful career in global financial journalism with the Financial Times in London.

I wasn't going to let the doctors defeat me. And that is the key to this book. Yes, it is an autobiography of sorts but it is not an ego trip. The purpose is to show that epilepsy can be seen by doctors, by sections of society and some families as a major obstacle to a person's progress through life. But it does not have to be that way.

With will and determination many of the negatives that can be associated with the condition can be overcome and people can have a successful career and life despite the many downsides of epilepsy. I have been very fortunate in my life to achieve many of my ambitions and achieve even more than that and while epilepsy has always been part of my life I have been able to overcome the downsides and in many ways it has strengthened me to achieve more.

In a strange way, having epilepsy has made me stronger and I can honestly say that I would not have been able to have the successes in my life and career without having my own personal struggle with epilepsy and, in particular, proving the doctors wrong.

My life and successful career is an example of what can be done despite the negative effects of epilepsy. Could I have predicted this outcome as a teenager struggling with severe seizures? Definitely not. But mine is an example of what can be done with will and determination and I hope the stories and anecdotes in this book can act as an example to those with the condition that all is possible. You don't have to allow the views and prejudices surrounding epilepsy to overcome you, it is possible to fight back. It is possible to turn the negatives of epilepsy into positives. This is what this book is about and I hope it can be a useful guide to what is possible.

It is not a comprehensive medical history of the condition, but at a time when more people are beginning to speak out about mental health issues after generations of silence and issues being swept under the carpet, it is my attempt to articulate my various experiences with epilepsy. It is also my hope that by talking openly about it, this may reduce some of the stigmas and misunderstandings surrounding the condition.

First, I want to outline the core structural issues encompassing epilepsy but as I am not a doctor or an academic, I am using information from the World Health Organisation to describe the key facts and then filling in some of the detail with my own personal stories. I enclose details from the World Health Organisation (WHO) along with some key facts in an appendix to this introduction.

APPENDIX

How does the World Health Organisation(WHO) describe epilepsy and its impact on the 50 million people worldwide with the disorder? I will include the basics described on the WHO's website. This is not a comprehensive listing but I hope its scale and diversity give some indication of the complexity and difficulties facing those 50 million people.

WHO Key Facts

- Epilepsy is a chronic noncommunicable disorder of the brain that affects people of all ages.

- Approximately 50 million people worldwide have epilepsy, making it one of the most common neurological diseases globally.

- Nearly 80% of the people with epilepsy live in low- and middle-income countries.

- People with epilepsy respond to treatment approximately 70% of the time.

- About three fourths of people with epilepsy living in low- and middle- income countries do not get the treatment they need.

- In many parts of the world, people with epilepsy and their families suffer from stigma and discrimination.

These Key Facts from the WHO provide a basic synopsis and I will add what I believe are a few relevant details from the WHO website that provide some core data to an understanding of the global condition.

"Epilepsy is a chronic disorder of the brain that affects people worldwide. It is characterized by recurrent seizures, which are brief episodes of involuntary movement that may involve a part of the body (partial) or the entire body (generalized), and are sometimes accompanied by loss of consciousness and control of bowel or bladder function.

Seizure episodes are a result of excessive electrical discharges in a group of brain cells. Different parts of the brain can be the site of such discharges. Seizures can vary from the briefest lapses of attention or muscle jerks to severe and prolonged convulsions. Seizures can also vary in frequency, from less than 1 per year to several per day."

"Approximately 50 million people currently live with epilepsy worldwide. The estimated proportion of the general population with active epilepsy (i.e. continuing seizures or with the need for treatment) at a given time is between 4 and 10 per 1000 people. However, some studies in low- and middle-income countries suggest that the proportion is much higher, between 7 and 14 per 1000 people.

Globally, an estimated 2.4 million people are diagnosed with epilepsy each year. In high-income countries, annual new cases are between 30 and 50 per 100 000 people in the general population. In low- and middle-income countries, this figure can be up to two times higher.

This is likely due to the increased risk of endemic conditions such as malaria or neurocysticercosis; the higher incidence of road traffic injuries; birth-related injuries; and variations in medical infrastructure, availability of preventative health programmes and accessible care. Close to 80% of people with epilepsy live in low- and middle-income countries."

"Epilepsy is not contagious. The most common type of epilepsy, which affects 6 out of 10 people with the disorder, is called idiopathic epilepsy and has no identifiable cause.

Epilepsy with a known cause is called secondary epilepsy, or symptomatic epilepsy. The causes of secondary (or symptomatic) epilepsy could be:

- brain damage from prenatal or perinatal injuries (e.g. a loss of oxygen or trauma during birth, low birth weight),

- congenital abnormalities or genetic conditions with associated brain malformations,

- a severe head injury,

- a stroke that restricts the amount of oxygen to the brain,

- an infection of the brain such as meningitis, encephalitis, neurocysticercosis,

- certain genetic syndromes,

- a brain tumor.

"Epilepsy accounts for 0.6%, of the global burden of disease, a time-based measure that combines years of life lost due to premature mortality and time lived in less than full health. Epilepsy has significant economic implications in terms of health care needs, premature death and lost work productivity.

Although the social effects vary from country to country, the discrimination and social stigma that surround epilepsy worldwide are often more difficult to overcome than the seizures themselves. People living with epilepsy can be targets of prejudice. The stigma of the disorder can discourage people from seeking treatment for symptoms, so as to avoid becoming identified with the disorder."

"People with epilepsy can experience reduced access to health and life insurance, a withholding of the opportunity to obtain a driving license, and barriers to enter particular occupations, among other limitations. In many countries legislation reflects centuries of misunderstanding about epilepsy. For example:

- In both China and India, epilepsy is commonly viewed as a reason for prohibiting or annulling marriages.

- In the United Kingdom, laws which permitted the annulment of a marriage on the grounds of epilepsy were not amended until 1971.

- In the United States of America, until the 1970s, it was legal to deny people with seizures access to restaurants, theatres, recreational centres and other public buildings.

These basic assessments from the WHO website provide a simple and core underpinning of the issues facing those with epilepsy and I firmly believe that the scale of epilepsy worldwide is not fully appreciated, the issues surrounding it could be much better understood by and conveyed to the public worldwide. There is a long way to go to improve the plight of the 50 million or more people worldwide with the condition.

In trying to understand my own epilepsy it is perhaps useful to examine why I have epilepsy and the type of tonic-clonic seizures I have had for the past 60 years. No doctor has ever tried to explain why I have epilepsy except to mention a number of possible causes and the short answer is I don't know why I have epilepsy and I am convinced I will never know.

Yes, I was six weeks premature at birth and that could have been a factor and yes, I fell off my trike at around five in the back yard which caused serious head injuries. This led to a two week stay in hospital. But apart from those two incidents no one can say for sure what led to my seizures and this is one of the frustrating aspects of the condition. No one knows with any degree of certainty, you just have to accept the condition without understanding why. This can be a major source of frustration for sufferers and their families.

In the final part of this introduction it is useful to explain why the four well known personalities were included on the cover. In a world that has often shunned the mention of the word epilepsy and cloaked the existence of the condition in all sorts of stigmas and prejudices these four, Julius Caesar, Joan of Arc, Fyodor Dostoyevsky and Vincent Van Gogh, all are understood to have suffered from epilepsy (although specifics are not well understood) but, nevertheless they managed to lead successful lives on the world stage.

Like epilepsy itself, these characters are wildly diverse from the Roman leader Julius Caesar over two thousand years ago to French heroine, Joan of Arc, in the 15th century to Russian writer, Fyodor Dostoyevsky in the 19th century along with Dutch artist Vincent Van Gogh, these famous personalities have made great contributions in their time despite having epilepsy. They showed that great achievements could be made in the face of the adversity of epilepsy and this is also the theme of this book, epilepsy need not be a hindrance to a successful life. These four did not have easy lives but despite their own health issues they made strong contributions in their fields. They are examples to follow.

I have used these four historical characters on the cover to reflect the achievements they have made while coping with epilepsy. This book is not about them as such and I do apologise to those who may expect to learn more about them. This book focuses on my experiences of epilepsy and my more modest stories related to my life.

Nevertheless, research is always good and while there are many famous people who have suffered from epilepsy this book is not about them. I could not resist, however, including a story about Dutch artist Vincent Van Gogh contained in a 2016 book by Bernadette Murphy entitled "Van Gogh's Ear - The True Story".

In a chapter entitled 'Troubled Genes', Ms Murphy includes the patient notes of Dr Theophile Peyron relating to Vincent Van Gogh on 9 May 1889. These notes are understood to be the only medical diagnosis available of Van Gogh's illness. The doctor's note below reflects many of the ambiguities and difficulties facing both those suffering from epilepsy and those trying to find solutions which apply equally well today in the 21st century. The complexity endures.

"I the undersigned, Doctor of Medicine, Director of the Saint- remy mental home, certify that the man named Vincent van Gogh, aged 36, a native of Holland and at present domiciled in Arles (Bouches-du-Rhone), underwent treatment at this city's infirmary, suffered an attack of acute mania with visual and auditory hallucinations that led him to mutilate himself by cutting off his ear. Today he appears to have regained his reason, but he does not feel he has the strength or the courage to live independently and has himself asked to be admitted to the home. Based on all the above, I consider that M. Van Gogh is subject to attacks of epilepsy, separated by long intervals, and that it is advisable to place him under long-term observation in the institution."

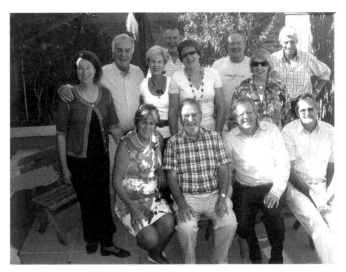

Monash mates in 2006
Back row, Lynn Dowling, Andrew Kennedy,Fiona Field, Tom Barrett,
Marg Renou, Pete Mahon, Chrissie Mahon, David Field.
Front row, Sue Barrett, Steve Timewell, Mike Dowling and Bill Renou

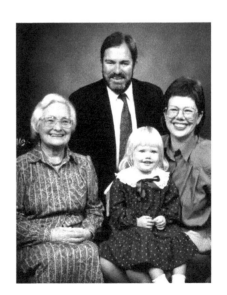

Granny and the Clocks in 1991
Left to right, Granny
Nora,Steve Timewell, Liberty
Timewell, Gail Timewell.

GROWING UP WITH EPILEPSY

I was 13 in 1964 when, to my knowledge, I had my first tonic- clonic seizure at the bus stop near home on the way to school. While I had heard the word epilepsy before, I knew nothing about the condition. All I had gleaned, if I knew anything, were some of the prejudices and misconceptions that had grown up over the centuries, the possession of devils, the danger of flashing lights and the overall fear the word engendered.

It was not something that was understood, like a broken arm, and as I and my family struggled to get a grip on what had happened at the bus stop I began to realise there were not a lot of readily digestible facts on the subject and there were no easy answers. Also, it was 1964 (The Beatles had just released "*I Wanna Hold Your Hand*"), the Internet and Wikipedia were four decades away and a young Australian schoolboy had no one to ask and no way to find out.

All I knew was that Dad was very upset, and Mum too, and, in the tradition of the era I was the last person to be told anything meaningful. Doctors were not much help either; while I knew my specialist, Dr Sewell, spoke to Dad more openly, I was not party to those conversations, I was kept in the dark.

This corresponded to the attitudes of the day where family secrets were kept hidden from younger members, family issues were not discussed openly and the fearful shroud that the word epilepsy evoked meant that Little Stephen's episodes, so to speak, were addressed in silence.

This silence in the family was emphasised particularly by a call

I made to my sister Julie (three years older) a few weeks after I started writing this book in January 2017. I asked my sister if she could remember my seizures and anything about them. I was trying to add some depth to my coverage but I found my sister's response quite a shock.

While I thought my first seizure was in 1964, over 50 years ago as I have said, Julie calmly told me I was having seizures 60 years ago when I was around five or so. She related a seizure down at the beach nearby where she and Dad dragged me out of the water and other seizures at home in the kitchen. I had no knowledge of any of this, certainly not the one at the beach.

My sister Julie related all this to a time I fell off my trike in the backyard, damaged my head and spent a couple of weeks in hospital. I must have been around five in 1956. I was aware of that and the stay in hospital but the word epilepsy was never mentioned nor the seizures that occurred in subsequent years.

Somewhat shocked by Julie's revelations to me I spoke to my older sister Margaret later in January 2017 and she confirmed the same story of my seizure at Park Street beach around 1956 and the issue of the trike accident. This was all amazing for me to hear in 2017, 60 years after it all began.

I asked Julie how she felt about seeing me have a seizure. She remembered being taken aback by it all but added somewhat calmly: "When we realised you recovered after a couple of hours sleep, we got used to it and just accepted it." No doubt Dad would have said not to mention it to me and she didn't, I was completely unaware of these childhood seizures and it was never mentioned when I went to my appointments with Dr Sinn aged seven. At that stage I started taking Dilantin (or Phenytoin as it is known today) but I thought it was because they said I was highly strung, whatever that meant.

Those calls in January 2017 helped explain why I was going to a specialist paediatrician for years and taking a medication that was described as an anti-depressant, whatever that was, and the connection with the trike accident now 60 years ago. But in the true style of the times nothing was explained to me. It has only become a little clearer in 2017, decades after these episodes.

Would it have been better if I had been told the truth by Dad and even by my sister? Sixty years on part of me says yes but, in hindsight and considering the culture of the day, I have to say it probably did not make much difference. I was looked after and loved at home and that was that. My sister did what she was told and I remained in the dark.

Some Background

I was born on 21st December 1950, the first child of Eileen (nee Cairns) Timewell. What I did not realise until I was seven or eight was that Dad had had a very sad and difficult life which was made more complicated by adhering to various aspects of secrecy which seemed part of the particular culture of the time.

I was blissfully unaware that Dad's first wife, Adelaide, who gave birth to sister Margaret in 1936, had the severe misfortune to die during the birth of my sister Julie in November 1947. With great help from Margaret, his mother (Grandma) and his sister (Aunty Valda) Dad managed to bring up Julie, run his various grain businesses and meet his second wife Eileen.

And then I came along in December 1950 and Julie and I both thought that Eileen was our mother. Somehow, our older sister Margaret was part of the conspiracy of silence and Julie and brother Stephen(me) continued in happy ignorance over what had actually happened. With this much family secrecy taking place it is no wonder that epilepsy did not represent a challenge in terms of disclosure or openness.

The 1950s were a positive time and I was very fortunate to have a loving family, loving parents and to be born at the beginning of the post-war boom. In the mid-1950s I was aware that something significant had happened to me in the back yard when I fell off my trike. I remember being in hospital for two weeks and it not being a pleasant experience.

In hindsight, did I have a seizure on my trike and land on my head or did I just land on my head? I don't know. Of course no one mentioned epilepsy and it has only been in 2017 that seizures on the beach and in the kitchen were mentioned. So I have no idea and until early 2017 I believed my first seizure was when I was 13, not earlier.

My understanding of my seizures, the trike incident and its aftermath were all completely overshadowed, however, by a more dramatic event that would dominate my future. In late 1956 Melbourne hosted the Olympics and like any good Aussie boy of five I was excited to go and I can still remember parts of it very clearly. We also bought our first TV for the Olympics, the first house in the street to have one, a 17inch Phillips, and everyone came to gawk and wonder at it. But I was not prepared for what happened in December after the Olympics.

Approaching Christmas and the summer holidays it was getting hotter. I can remember Margaret had prepared a usual dinner of lamb chops, peas and mashed potatoes and then Dad came in very upset and beckoned Margaret to the hall, Julie and I stayed eating in the kitchen.

Julie and I wondered what was wrong and went up to see Dad and Margaret. They were crying dramatically and it was not good. Dad said to me: "Mum would not be coming home again," and so began a desperately bad time in my life. It was a blunt reshaping of my previous beautiful world. I was five turning six and my mother had just died, something to do with kidney failure. Decades later that problem could have been solved easily with dialysis but in 1956 the technology did not exist and my Mum was gone.

The next few weeks went by in a blur, it was the summer school holidays and the reality of Mum's passing was very painful. For Dad and Margaret it was their second wife/mother to die in nine years, although neither Julie nor I knew that then. In February 1957 Julie and I started school again and for want of a better term we just got on with it. Getting on with it was what we did, we had no choice. Did we have proper time to grieve, whatever that means? The answer is probably not, but unlike Dad and Margaret it was new for Julie and I, we were very alone and all I could do was cry myself to sleep every night.

For Dad and Margaret they had to get on with it too. Survival was everything. It was a tough time. I suppose it made me stronger in many ways but I did not really understand what that meant then. I wanted my Mum and as Dad said, she wasn't coming home again. But Dad, Margaret and Julie were still there and I was loved, life carried on.

The next year or two continued, I remember missing my Mum a lot, but in typical fashion nobody spoke about it and life went on in its own bubble. The next big event was my big sister Margaret getting engaged and then married in October 1958 to John Fleming, who also went to my school, Xavier College, and was a real big brother to me. I idolised him and I was always desperate to kick the footy with him when he came down to Park Street. Margaret's wedding at home in the back garden was a tremendous family occasion which I can still remember in detail, especially the ice cream dessert, and I suppose this opened a new chapter in my life.

In late December that year, around my birthday, there was another wedding, Dad married Helena Murnane in Carlton opposite our beloved Carlton Football Ground. Dad had obviously courted Helena (or Nana Helen as I now refer to her) for the previous year or so but I was probably unaware of the details and the significance of it all. Dad had wanted a mother for Julie and me and a companion for himself. Julie and I understood this but had no knowledge that this was Dad's third marriage; we were probably the only ones to not know Dad's full marital history and the burden he carried with the deaths of both Adelaide and Eileen.

Nana Helen was an excellent lady who was very good to Julie and I, but after the wedding we had to call her something. It was an interesting change for Julie and me and brought forward an important philosophical debate. In my mind I wanted a Mum and, although young (just 8), I well understood if I wanted her to be my Mum I had to call her Mum and that is what I decided to do. Julie was three years older than me and for whatever reasons she was reluctant to call her Mum and called her Helen. In hindsight this was a wise decision on my part and my relationship with my new 'Mum' was very good.

I was a somewhat sickly child with many colds, asthma and flus and I missed a lot of school when I was seven. In grade 4 at age 8 Mum and I decided to keep a calendar of sick days and I also started riding my new bike to school, a couple of miles away, with Freddie Tiernan. For whatever reason I did not miss a day's school in 1959 and I became healthier and was unaware of any seizures, if they did happen.

I was a very fortunate little boy, I had a new Mum, I was healthier and we spent a lot of time in the country at Creswick, 60 miles out of Melbourne where Mum's aging parents lived. We were a fully functioning family again, Julie and I would go out and help at Dad's dog biscuit business in Mont Albert and his grain business in Burnley and a lot of time was spent in the country with new relatives and activities.

As I was finishing at the Xavier preparatory school, Kostka Hall, when I was 11 and 12 I was the biggest boy in the class and because I was so big I became a star at football. All we did was play cricket and football and go to the beach or pool. I was also very worried about being kept down at school so I always studied very hard and was always in the Top 10 of our 40-boy class. In grade 8 in 1963 I starred at football (Aussie Rules of course) and to make sure I made it to the senior school I studied as much as I could and finished 4th in the class and received a state scholarship. I regularly kept seeing Dr Sinn for check-ups and kept taking my pills, the side effect of which was to make me quite hairy and I started to shave early, which I thought was good. There was no mention of any seizures.

And so I lived through those years from five to 13, having an unknown number of seizures, being attended to by Dr Sinn and being blissfully unaware of what was wrong with me.

All that changed completely at the bus stop in 1964 when I was 13. Something significant had happened. I had badly damaged myself and lost some teeth, it could not be hidden any longer. The cat was out of the bag. My family seemingly had known for years there was a problem but now I had to come to terms with the fact that I had epilepsy, whatever that meant.

Yes, around the kitchen table the family discussed that Dad would drive me and others to school to avoid any further bus stop incidents but we did not discuss what had happened at the bus stop. My sister Julie (three years older) was aware of the issue but we did not discuss epilepsy as such and my friends in the street were probably aware that something was wrong but it was never mentioned. We just continued to do what young teenagers did in those days, play football in the winter (Aussie Rules of course), cricket in the summer and spend a lot of time on the beach which was a mere 100 yards from home.

My secondary education at Xavier College, one of the top Melbourne private schools continued as usual. I was not aware that teachers knew anything about my seizures which occurred regularly in 1964 but I was exempted from compulsory school cadets (military training) on Monday (on Dad's intervention) and I was hugely pleased about that. No one liked cadets. One key element of my introduction to epilepsy was that all my seizures in the first year or more were at home before school and in the following four years of my secondary education I never had a seizure at school and therefore my epilepsy never attracted the attention and exposure it would have or could have otherwise.

I was never teased or bullied at school and being one of the biggest boys in the class and in the Under14A football team, epilepsy never impacted on my social and sporting life. Also, I was in the top academic class of four classes in my year and that continued throughout school and despite the advent of seizures in 1964 I continued to be in the top half of the top class for the next two years and beyond. Did my teachers know? I was not aware they did, and did not feel any preferential treatment in class or on the playing fields.

In essence my initial exposure to epilepsy was relatively mild, and although I had severe tonic-clonic seizures with no warning signs at all I was fortunate to always have them early in the morning before going to school with minimum public disruption or exposure. I had probably around 15 seizures in 1964 and

1965 but without great damage, only the odd tooth loss and badly bitten tongue. When I had a seizure I just stayed home, slept it off, and next day was back to school and no one else was aware.

The real problem came later in 1964 when my specialist Dr Sewell took me aside and explained what the future held for me. I had considerable experience in seeing specialists as from about seven years of age Dad took me to see Dr Sinn, a paediatrician. I was told that I was highly strung and hence was required to take a drug called dilantin (today's name is phenytoin) to calm me down. I never felt I needed calming down but, certainly in the 1950s, you did as you were told and just accepted it. Curiously, as a teenager, I continued to be prescribed Dilantin, and I then understood it was an anti-epilepsy medication.

I was well used to taking pills and going to my regular appointments in Collins Street, Melbourne with specialists Dr Sinn and then Dr Sewell, Dad's specialist as well. But I was shocked one day in 1964 when Dr Sewell outlined what I could not do in my life ahead.

He told me bluntly that I could not expect to finish school, I could not expect to go to university and while I knew by then that I could not expect to get a driver's licence I was alarmed that my academic prospects were written off in one fell swoop.

Till this day I don't know why Dr Sewell told me this in such a brutal way. In more recent years I wondered whether he wanted to stir me up, presenting the worst case scenario first and forcing me to lift my game. In the 21st century doctors have been surprised by his grim approach and tone then, but it did have the impact of making me hugely determined to prove him wrong. I was determined to finish school and go to university and Dr Sewell was not going to stop me.

The short answer is I did finish school at Xavier College, gained a Bachelor of Economics at Monash University in 1971 and in 1982 a Masters in Islamic History and Arabic from the University of Chicago and in 2017 I am Editor Emeritus of The Banker magazine, part of the Financial Times Group in London. Neither Dr Sewell nor my father lived long enough to see all that but I am hugely pleased to have proved Dr Sewell wrong and proved that my epilepsy was not a hindrance to a successful and fulfilling life. But in 1964 I did not know what lay ahead and at that time the prognosis did not look good.

Dad continued to worry about me as the seizures continued but in 1965 he tried a new strategy. Chiropractors were new in Melbourne and this fellow in St Kilda Road, near the old St Kilda Football Ground, ventured that he could straighten my bent spine and perhaps help my epilepsy. We gave it a try and for a year or more Dad would pick me up from school twice a week after school and we would go to St Kilda where they endeavoured to straighten my spine.

Did this have any impact? After a year or more of this chiropractor hammering my spine twice a week, he showed me an X-ray of a spine, much straighter than the original and believed to be my spine. I, of course, felt no different but, to be fair, in the course of the year or more of sessions the frequency of my seizures declined. Was it the chiropractor who helped my seizures decline or was it just a coincidence? I will never know the answer but Dad was pleased, I was pleased and I was going into my last two years of school.

The seizures continued but their frequency diminished and I carried on studying hard, playing football and doing all that normal teenagers did in the 1960s. It was a great time to be alive, I had a very loving family and the dreaded word epilepsy, which had put a cloud over my life, appeared to be diminishing. I kept doing well academically at school (or sticking it to Dr Sewell) and I was determined not to let epilepsy get me down. I had many advantages in my life, good parents, good family and good school and I was not going to let epilepsy slow me down.

And so I progressed to Leaving (5th Year) and then Matriculation (Final Year) and while I still kept having seizures though at a decreasing frequency I just got on with my life, put epilepsy in the background and focussed on proving Dr Sewell wrong. Unlike the 21st century with greater access to more information and the Internet etc there was no one to ask in the 1960s, Dad was doing his best and I just had to get on with it, there was no choice.

I seemed to be good at exams at school and while there was a lot of pressure to succeed and go to university I was used to the stress and all this did not necessarily cause more seizures. I worked hard and just got on with it. Another advantage I had was that my parents did not put expectations on me. Dad was just pleased if I kept breathing and although school had high expectations of what we would achieve I had no pressure at home. I would have been the first in our family to go to university anyway. So I studied hard and pushed myself and with good teachers at school I achieved the academic results to allow me to go to my first choice, Economics and Politics at Monash University.

I was thrilled and so were Mum and Dad. I did enjoy telling Dr Sewell at my next appointment and received a bland reaction. I had got through school and made it to university with no particular help from Dr Sewell.

In looking back on those years should I have sought different advice, done things differently? The answer is perhaps yes but this was the 1960s, the sources of information available today did not exist then, the institutional help was not there such as Epilepsy Action. Attitudes to epilepsy often harked back to the dark days of the past where it was not well understood medically and generally misinterpreted, with some suggesting it was linked to possession by devils or similar bogus speculation.

In hindsight I was fortunate under the circumstances to have done as well as I did. Mum and Dad did well to steer me through and it is important to stress that my epilepsy in those days was well controlled compared with many other people and my seizures, although I had no warning, were always early in the morning and not overly dangerous. I was very lucky in my experience with epilepsy but it did impact on my life.

With the condition now affecting 50 million people worldwide and with over 40 different types of epilepsy now diagnosed, it is important to better understand the diverse impact of the condition on those afflicted so that better support can be given to both patients and their families.

GETTING THROUGH UNIVERSITY WITH EPILEPSY

1968 was an important year politically across the globe, revolutions, the Vietnam War and massive social changes dominated and a young Xavier College schoolboy from Brighton, just 17, was beginning an economics degree at Monash in March. I had wanted to go into business, like my father, and I believed economics was the best grounding possible, so I combined economics with a second major in accounting. I was quite good at mathematics at school and also included that in my first year with mandatory economic statistics making up my initial four courses.

March 1968, almost fifty years ago today, was a critical time for me in my development. I did not know what the future held for me and the world was changing dramatically. All I knew was that I wanted to be a part of it. I was young and naïve, as we probably all were, and I was very sociable, partying and pubbing as much as possible. I had a lot of friends in Brighton from a variety of schools and from Xavier and, although I was relatively young, it was an easy transition from life based around school and Brighton to one at Monash, a few miles away. As opposed to students in the US moving interstate to college or British students going to university in other parts of the country I was going just a few miles to Monash in an outer suburb of Melbourne and all the travel and social networks were much the same as in school days.

The changes were not that dramatic at all, we had had plenty of contact with girls in Brighton, university represented, in a sense, a big new party and play area where we were expected to do some work and learn something. Unlike other countries, most students in Melbourne lived at home when they first went to university and so life was not that radically different. And so it was for me. And while I was well aware of my epilepsy, university did not present any particularly new challenges as long as my seizures remained in the early morning as they did.

Monash represented 'Halcyon' days for my generation then. We believed that all things were possible, and as a young Australian they were. There were important global social and economic issues going on but for baby-boomers (born after the end of World War II) like me and my colleagues it was a perfect time to be alive and we absorbed it all in a ferociously hedonistic way. Being called up to fight in the Vietnam war was a downside but I managed to avoid that and we just enjoyed socialising, drinking and doing some work, we were lucky people in what has been described as 'The Lucky Country' of Australia.

Did epilepsy impinge on my social and academic life at Monash? I will discuss transport later, but did I discuss my epilepsy with friends, were they aware that I had seizures and what were their views? In many ways I fudged this question and while I did not hide the fact that I had epilepsy I did not labour it either. My good Monash friend Dee Austin (then Dee Collie), who 50 years later lives near me in London, along with good pals Mike Dowling and Pete Mahon, were all well aware of my epilepsy but neither I nor they made a big deal of it, it was not a subject of conversation at the pub. Yes it was possible that my epilepsy came up as a reason why I did not drive a car, as Pete noted, but once mentioned that was that and I just carried on and led a very normal life. In asking friends about this period they seemed to accept it and made no fuss. They acknowledged Steve had epilepsy but were not bothered by it. Steve's epilepsy was basically irrelevant to their lives. Dee did mention that on Saturday's when we met to go to the football at the Melbourne Cricket Ground (MCG) I did not show at times and that was due to a seizure in the morning. I don't remember those occasions but I did make the MCG on many other occasions.

I did not talk about it and neither did they. Like school, I never had seizures during the day at university and so the harsh reality of witnessing me having a seizure did not occur. In the time- honoured way I had lived my life up to that date my university life just continued and my seizures, if and when I had them, I did not let them interfere in my social or academic life. While I remember still taking dilantin (now called phenytoin) while at university, I believe I was on a relatively low dose of one or two per day compared to four a day in 2017, I was relatively well-controlled in the doctor-speak of the time.

Transport was a critical issue in such a large place like Melbourne and when I started at Monash I was still too young for a driver's licence at 18 and I knew my epilepsy would preclude me from ever getting a licence. So how did I get around in a large city with relatively little in the way of public transport? One managed a lot of lifts from friends to make the nine mile trek to Monash but necessity is the mother of invention and so I started hitch hiking and this proved to be a great bonus for me, not only at Monash but over the following 15 years in Australia and the US. In the late 1960s and early 1970s hitch hiking was a relatively normal activity for young people although its popularity had faded by the 1980s.

As a relatively well-off middle class student most of my colleagues would somehow acquire an old Mini or Beetle when they passed their driving test but although Dad would have given me a car, as he did my sister, that was not going to happen for me. Hitch hiking was my way forward and it proved to be a great education for me in many ways. I was not going to let my epilepsy affect me and although I couldn't drive I found a way around it and hitching was the vehicle.

I remember well after a few years of hitching I decided to hitch from Melbourne to Perth to see some cousins. Dad, not surpisingly, was not a great advocate of hitching but he knew there were few alternatives. I will always remember his sad face as he dropped me at the edge of Melbourne at the start of my 3,000 mile epic journey. If I hadn't had epilepsy I would never have got into hitch hiking and I would never have had the myriad of strong and worthwhile experiences that hitching brought both at home and abroad. I did not realise then that I would never have had the confidence to hitch hike across America in summer 1971 if hitching had not been an important part of my life at university.

I must add that I did do more than just drinking and hitching at Monash. I did study and work hard, and although I probably averaged four seizures a year at university they were in the morning and they did not impact on my academic or social performance. I was not a brilliant student but I worked hard and managed to get through. I was just a good average student who had a wide circle of friends, as I always had, and achieved my Bachelor of Economics in 1971 with two long summer vacations working as an auditor with the global accounting firm now known as Ernst & Young. Also, I became President of Monash Golf Club and managed to organise an Australia-wide Intervarsity Golf Tournament in Melbourne in 1980 which was deemed a great success. My Monash mates were a key part of my life and I still keep in touch with many of them almost 50 years later. Although I live in London today one of my Monash mates lives not far away in Islington and many use our London residence as a staging post on European visits.

My university years were uneventful from an epilepsy perspective. Seizures continued but did not seriously impact on me. Epilepsy by accident got me involved in hitch hiking for which I am hugely grateful. As I have often said, out of all bad comes good and I have been fortunate enough to have learnt that lesson many times in my life.

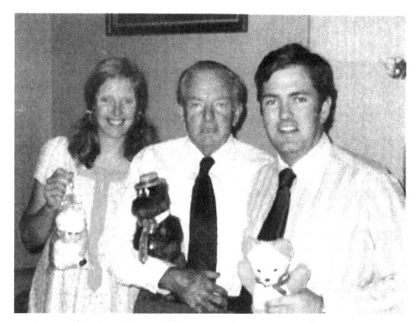

Sister Julie, Steve Timewell Senior and Steve Timewell Junior c1971.

TRAVELLING THE WORLD AFTER UNIVERSITY

In July 1971 I had planned to go on a world trip with my sister Julie who was then a trained nurse. Like many young Australians we were keen to see the world and also well aware that while Australia offered many advantages we knew the world was out there to be discovered. Unfortunately for me she decided to get married in March. Nevertheless, I still decided to go off, but now I was going on my own when I graduated.

While most of my Monash mates headed for the job market I was transfixed by travelling the world and absorbing it all first hand. My key objective was to stand in Moscow's Red Square as well as trying to see all the places in the US and Europe I had heard so much about down under. Little did I know when I planned to hitch hike across the US and head on to Europe in July 1971 that I would spend over 40 of the next 45 years or more overseas, living in Egypt, the US and London and visiting and writing about over 60 countries across the globe. I did have a lot of travel ambitions and in hindsight I have managed to achieve and surpass them all.

But in July 1971 it was all out there and ahead of me. I also had huge support at home, both financially and personally. Dad and my new Mum were always very supportive and although I knew they were worried about me travelling on my own they did not stand in my way. I was excited and nervous as I flew to San Francisco via Hawaii on the first leg of my global tour. I was on my own but I was not afraid of my epilepsy, I knew I just had to overcome my fear and any problems I might have. I was not going to let epilepsy spoil my adventures and my new education post-university.

Landing at San Francisco Airport brought a new cold reality, I was on my own at the start of an amazing adventure. And so I hitch hiked out of the airport and headed for Berkeley which was the centre of the flower-power movement and the place to be in the 1970s for music, drugs and just about everything. I managed to hitch into Berkeley without too much trouble thanks to my years of experience hitching in Melbourne, and following my strategy of targeting fraternity houses for my places to stay I walked into a fraternity house in the university area and I was away.

To my surprise I was an instant hit the moment I opened my mouth and they took in my Aussie accent and there I was in the summer of 1971 in California taking everything in, having no trouble finding a bed (for free) and going from one party to another. I had with me a copy of a well known book *"The US on a Dollar a Day"*, this was my hitch hiker's guide and it worked a treat. I stayed a while in Berkeley taking in the fun scene, my fill of hot dogs and beer and then I thought I should move on. My greatest problem was that all the young people in the world, it seemed, were hitching and it was hard to find a reasonable spot at the side of the road to put out your thumb.

Nevertheless, it was not too difficult and I soon found myself in San Jose and San Jose State University where the fraternity houses again provided a ready source of friends, parties and easy accommodation. I was having a ball and lifts were fun too, it seemed I could do no wrong.

I headed on south to Los Angeles and while I had to cope with getting dropped in a bad black neighbourhood I found my way to Hollywood where I worked painting a house for a while for one of my Disney childhood idols, Cheryl, from the Mouseketeers. Great fun. I then started the long haul east where I discovered I had a frightening fear of heights at the Grand Canyon. Being drawn to jump off those cliffs was no fun but reaching Las Vegas and seeing Dionne Warwick live for $10 was a huge treat which I will always remember.

Hitching was great fun and full of surprises. Further east I was picked up by a genuine Wichita lineman heading to Wichita, it was surreal beyond my wildest dreams. Despite all this excitement, of a sort, I had no seizures and felt terrific and kept on heading east across mid-America until I reached Ohio. After over 45 years the details are a bit hazy but I was heading for Sharon, Pennsylvannia, where the sister of my best Brighton mate, Freddie Tiernan, had stayed as an exchange student years before.

Getting there was very strange as I got picked up by a group of black guys who used me as a white stooge at a series of gas stations passing off fake gemstones as the real thing. The ruse worked for them and I got to Sharon where Gini Tiernan's US family gave me a wonderful American experience with lots of basketball and incredible hamburgers. They also suggested I work on a summer camp as a volunteer in neighbouring Ohio and so for a month I stayed on a magnificent country farm, playing Carole King's 'Tapestry' album and entertaining loads of teenagers on summer camp. It could not have been more fun or more enjoyable.

A friend at the camp, Bob, asked me back to his home in Youngstown, Ohio, another decaying steel town, and a curious incident occurred which gave a new dimension to my hitching experience. As a young Australian on the road Bob wanted me to go on a local talk-back radio programme and amazingly enough the programme asked listeners to call in and offer the Aussie a lift to my next destination, Boston. Lots of offers came in and within a day or two I was on my way to Boston with a new family and my first experience of hitching by radio.

My radio family dropped me in Boston at the Massachusetts Institute of Technology (MIT) and I tried to find a place to stay. I had made it to the east coast and after some days touring Boston and the Cape Cod holiday area nearby I headed on my final US leg to New York and then on to Europe. Meanwhile I struggled to find a place to stay in Boston and settled on a couch in one of the reception buildings at MIT, not fancy but doable and a fine address.

Somehow I hitched my way to New York and ended up in the Bronx in a place that appeared safe. I was fortunate that no harm came my way, except perhaps in Los Angeles, and I was a good tourist in New York, seeing as much as I could and arranging my flight to London on a wet Friday night. Given my limited budget I was hugely pleased that my US adventure (including Dionne Warwick) had only cost $110 over the nine week period, incredibly cheap by 21st century standards. And so on to Europe, I had not visited all the US places I had thought about but I had seen a lot, done a lot and for only $110, it was a great trip so far.

Did I have any seizures in my venture across the US on my own? To my knowledge I had no seizures and I was not taking any medication. I felt I was seizure-free at this time for no apparent reason and not taking medication did not appear to cause any problems. Perhaps stupidly I ignored all the lessons of my life so far, ignored taking pills and it did not seem to have any impact. I was young, travelling and perhaps very lucky. The usual signs of a damaged tongue and drowsiness were not there and I just carried on oblivious.

Hitting London was key for a boy who had been brought up in a very Anglophile culture, it was hugely exciting but I was also aware of how much there was to do and my limited funds. I was quickly finding my way around the Monopoly board and taking in the historical monuments and cultural icons, it was fabulous. And then I got really lucky.

Somewhere near the British Museum I walked into a tourist travel shop and met a group of people planning a trip around Europe on an open-top double-decker bus. The itinerary went via Scandinavia to Russia and Moscow and then down to Istanbul and then back to London via Greece, Italy, France, Spain, Morocco and back up across the English Channel. It sounded terrific, touching base in all the places I wanted to see, including Moscow and at a price I could afford. But I had to decide then as the bus was off in a few days for this three month plus amazing journey. Not surprisingly I signed up on the spot, the last to do so and I was off.

Aussies are fearless travellers and it was no surprise that at least half the 24 people on Magnus, the double-decker, were Aussies. Rob Brown and Richard owned the bus, a converted RouteMaster, and were its drivers too, on this first time adventure that involved camping in tents (except in Russia) and seeing as much as we could across all of Europe. It was an amazing experience, 24 young girls and boys in good hippie tradition gallivanting across Europe, listening to the The Moody Blues album *'A Question of Balance'* all the time and absorbing all that Europe and the Seventies had to offer. Wow.

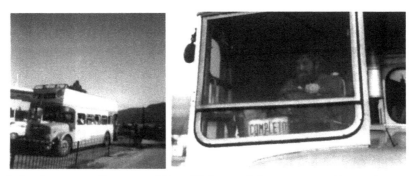

Double decker bus trip in Europe and Steve T. driving Magnus on pan-Europe bus trip, c 1971

The memories from those few months were huge, driving Magnus into Red Square and getting chased out by police, getting bogged in the Ukraine and managing to convince a farmer, who thought we were from outer space, to pull us out, enjoying Istanbul and the Bosphorus, the highlights were too numerous to mention. On returning to France from Spain Magnus was on his last legs and I stayed on the French coast while Rob went back to England with the crew for spare parts. By December our glorious tour was over but all of us met again in North London for my 21st birthday with massive quantities of Watney's Red Barrel and huge revelry.

Like my US travels, my European travels did not contain any adverse epilepsy stories. I knew my pals on the bus extremely well and they were aware of my epilepsy but no one, including me, made a fuss about it. To my knowledge I did not have any seizures on the three-month adventure, I led a totally normal life, and I just got on with enjoying the tour undaunted by anything.

In late December it was now dark and cold in England and I had little money left so reluctantly I thought of the warm Down Under at Christmas and decided to head home via Singapore and landed in Melbourne at the end of 1971 after a fabulous six months abroad, no medical problems and a mountain of memories.

Little did I realise then that I would only stay in Australia for the next five years and then I would live abroad and travel for the next 40 years or more. Travelling was in my blood and in 2017 it still continues to be a dominant part of my life. My post-university travels taught me an enormous amount and that time in the US and Europe were critical in building my confidence, my understanding of the world and its ways and in focusing on what I would do in the future. I was determined to achieve but had no idea what that meant and what form it would take. Returning to Melbourne was perhaps premature, I could have stayed away and travelled a lot more but being back home was not a bad place to be and created many more new opportunities, I was 21 and had a lot to do with my life.

As for epilepsy, it was not on my radar. To my knowledge my whole US and European venture involved no seizures at all and I had no source of medication. Was it possible that I survived all this travel and excitement without medication and seizures? To my knowledge the answer is definitely yes. This applies to further periods in my life where I was not aware of having either medication or seizures.

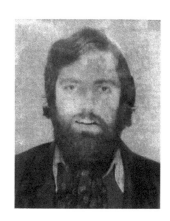

In my hippy days in 1971.

MY FIRST JOB AND MY ENTREPRENEURIAL YEARS

Back in Melbourne at the end of 1971 after my travel adventure in the US and Europe it was important not only to touch base with my family but also to get a job and genuinely begin my working career. I had a good economics degree from Monash University and, unlike the job market four and five decades on, there was at that time strong demand for graduates.

While I was enjoying the warm Aussie summer in January 1972 I was also looking hard for a graduate job and compared to the 21st century it was not too difficult. I did not know specifically what I wanted but I knew that it was not a job in accounting. At university I had two summer vacation jobs with one of the Big Four accounting firms, now known as Ernst & Young, and that was enough to convince me I did not want to continue being an auditor and become a chartered accountant, it was too boring as I saw it then. My good friend, Mike Dowling, went down that route but I was looking for something different and after a few weeks of applications and interviews I was offered a graduate appointment at Colonial Mutual Life on the princely sum of around A$5,000 per year to work on pension management and what they called in Australia at the time superannuation plans. A$5000 salary was competitive for 1972 so I could not complain.

By early February I had started work at CML in the heart of the City of Melbourne and I was away. While I was aware that I had a history of epilepsy it did not surface in the interviews and it passed without trace. Although I was young and enthusiastic what I was asked to do was paralysingly boring and on reflection I seemed to spend more time on arranging my social life than doing anything particularly productive on the insurance front. It became more interesting in time but while CML provided adequately for my drinking and socialising with lots of good mates it was rather dull and I was looking to see what I could do.

My sister was married in March 1971 and her husband, Tom Ericksen, provided a lot of excitement in his mixed business of private detective, repossession agent for the ANZ Bank and deal maker. I had not experienced anything like it and rightly or wrongly I was drawn in to some of his activities in my spare time. It was exciting and I was just 21 and Tom's was a whole new world. While my social life blossomed with constant parties, the Mitre Tavern after work and plenty of golf and going to the Melbourne Cricket Ground with my Dad and mates to the footy, I was not particularly enjoying CML but it was a job and a salary.

In 1972, epilepsy was not a problem for me and I believed I could make a contribution in this area. Epilepsy was not well understood and plenty of support was needed, I thought I would try to help. Without too much effort I became a board member of the Epilepsy Foundation of Victoria (the Melbourne equivalent of Epilepsy Action) and I was involved in various fund-raising activities. One such event was selling stick-on tattoos at the famous Sunbury Rock Festival outside Melbourne. We literally sold thousands of tattoos, raising awareness of epilepsy amongst young people. Over 45 years later I am now on the board of the British Epilepsy Association (known as Epilepsy Action), based in Leeds, and still looking for ways to raise awareness.

In 1973 a dramatic change occurred. Tom, my brother-in-law, was always the deal maker and Dad was keen to set up his 'little boy' in business just as his father had done with him. Tom spied an opportunity, the chance to buy a big coastal pub at Barwon Heads, not far from the family holiday home at Point Lonsdale. Dad bought into the idea and although none of us had ever run a big pub, Tom, the consummate salesman, convinced us that we could do it with me fronting the operation.

So in March 1973 we bought the Barwon Heads Hotel, which today remains an iconic feature of the coast, and I left CML to become a publican, young and enthusiastic but ignorant of running such a business and all the financial issues involved.

Tom's 'Donald Trump approach' had ignored some basics and while we sold a huge amount of beer over the next three or more years we had not appreciated that we were under-capitalised from the beginning, we had to take on a huge amount of debt and due to the 1973 global oil crisis my second mortgage went to over 20%. We sold a lot of beer and I learnt a lot about running such a business but all our profits went into paying off debt.

Not surprisingly by 1976 we had gone broke. Dad had died in mid- 1975 and I was accused of worrying him to death, which was not entirely true but the pub saga had not helped his health. I had had an intense business education in the pub and had failed dismally, I was 25 and had probably kept the pub going too long. Even the breweries that supported me said I should have gone broke earlier.

As far as epilepsy goes, I had plenty of stress but this did not turn into seizures and so during this 'pub' period I do not remember having any seizures during that time. Since I was no longer under Dr Sewell I had no regular medical attention and did not take medication for epilepsy or anything else. Why I dropped out of medication I cannot say in 2017, around 40 years later, but I was seizure-free and medication-free and I was in my mid-20s, again I was fortunate my health stayed steady.

Anyway, 1976 was a desperate time for us all, the pub was disposed of and in November 1976 in a very complex episode I got on a plane bound for London but instead I got off in Cairo, Egypt and I decided to build my new life there. My life back in Australia had been dramatic and eventful, I was under a huge amount of stress as the pub went broke and Dad died and our family fell apart. I was at the centre of it all and do not absolve myself of responsibility but I had to move on after this disaster and I did. It was tough but I was young and my health, or at least my epilepsy, was not holding me back.

MY YEARS ABROAD –
MY CAREER AND MY FAMILY

I left Australia in November 1976 and, although I have visited often I have not lived there since. I had to rebuild my life after the disaster in the pub venture at Barwon Heads which helped destroy my family's financial infrastructure and many family relationships as well.

It was not a happy period for me, I was down and out, but Cairo helped raise my spirits and my Egyptian experience from late 1976 to autumn 1980 put me back on course. Taking in the breadth of Egypt, trying to understand its huge diversity and its massive history was a life-changing event for me.

From being a rich, middle class Aussie youth who had somehow squandered his legacy I was now alone in an impoverished country trying to find my way. Not that I knew it when I arrived, Egypt would provide an unparalleled education for me in life, humanity and religion. I learned an enormous amount about the world in my new life as a teacher and later as a journalist. I was poor when I got there and still poor when I left but I was rich in personal experiences and rich in understanding.

My time there changed my life and while I had some dreadful times, with some linked to epilepsy, Egypt provided me with a catalyst and lessons that remain with me 40 years later; lessons that have provided the backbone of my life.

Egypt taught me, if I needed to be taught, that there were always people worse off than me and in a more desperate state than I could ever imagine. No matter how bad things may have looked for me at certain times I could always see where I lived and worked many Egyptians in a far worse state than I could ever be. And what made this lesson even more important was the attitude they showed. Egyptians were calm in the face of adversity and calamities and their good nature, kindness and humility enabled them to overcome all their problems with a smile. This for me is the lesson of Egypt that continues to sustain me and does not allow me to succumb when adversity strikes in its many forms.

In late November 1976 I got off the plane in Egypt and decided I would make my new start there rather than in London which I had been to five years before. I knew it was tough in London and thought I could make it better in Cairo. I got settled and got a job in a secondary school on my second day but lost it on my third, I was learning that Cairo could be tough too. With some luck and help I found an Armenian family to live with in the centre of town and I soon found a new English teaching job at Victoria College in Maadi, south of Cairo proper. It was all new and at school they handed me a copy of *Pride & Prejudice* and told me to get on with it. And so I did.

Teaching was a revelation to me and I loved it and somehow my mixed class of 13-14 year olds liked Mr Steve's unorthodox style and I relished the opportunity of such a completely different environment. From publican and private detective to teaching Jane Austin, it was a massive change. I did not have the fear, drama and threats of Australia, now I was surrounded by smiling young faces who wanted to learn and I surprised myself by being able to teach, at least better than I thought possible.

I loved the school bus, the kids and in the early days I added to my income through private lessons which generally included a much-needed meal. I was surviving more than well and the fear of repaying debt at the pub was replaced by fear of getting my lessons right. I was loving Cairo and its rich history, I learnt a lot from the multi-lingual Armenian family but moved on to stay in a little hotel, The Minerva, in the centre of town which became my home for almost the next four years.

After a few months I needed to boost my income and thought the local English language newspaper, The Egyptian Gazette, founded in 1880, badly needed some subbing and may need some help. I was welcomed with open arms and on 15 May 1977 I started in the evening around 6pm in another move that would change my life and introduce me to a career in journalism which lives on 40 years later.

On my first day I met my new boss Ramez al-Halawani and an Englishman Martin Rose, the latter became my best man ten years later in London and both are fine friends 40 years on. After putting the paper to bed we would invariably go down to the local watering holes for a few beers and some fine times were had with a hugely enjoyable crew.

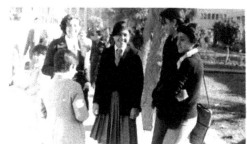

My students at Victory College, c 1977

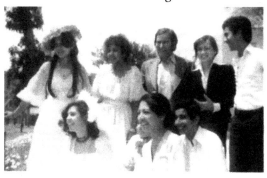

Cast of 'M Fair Lady' at Victory College c1978

Having broken my neck, with Martin Rose, Frances Matthew and Arnold Rose, c1978

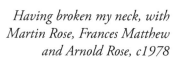

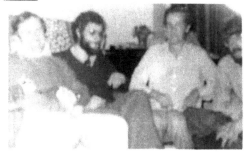

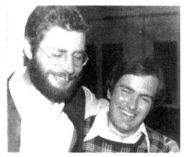

Martin Rose and Steve T. in Cairo in happy times, c1978

I was finding my feet, I was getting involved in the politics of the region and in journalism, and in a modest way I was paying my way in totally new careers. And, curiously, despite the new stresses I was seizure free and, for better or worse, medicine free too. I had no doctor and no pills.

Late 1977 caused some excitement both politically and medically. Egypt's President Sadat decided to go to Israel and I was chosen to go with him representing *The Egyptian Gazette*. It was an amazing experience for me, making the first telephone call ever from Israel to Egypt to report my findings was ground-breaking but I also created a near international incident when I had a seizure near the Dead Sea and Israeli officials were terrified that an 'Egyptian' journalist would die in one of their hospitals (see Epilepsy Action story). I recovered in hospital and the Israelis breathed a sigh of relief.

Back in Cairo I received a call from my family in Melbourne asking me, for various reasons, to move to Syria. I did not want to leave Cairo and I called on my friend Martin Rose to have a few beers to figure out what to do. The morning after (as detailed in another EA story) I had a seizure on my motor bike on my way to school, hit a tree and broke my neck.

The accident dramatically changed my life but with luck and good friends I stayed alive, did not go to Syria and in 1978 managed to take 16 of my school children to the UK on a school trip and saw some doctors in Edinburgh during the visit about my neck. While I remained in a dangerous and fragile condition I returned to Cairo and saved up for the operation in Scotland a year later where they would break my neck again and make it stable.

The operation had other consequences. While recuperating after the operation a friend pushed me into applying for a scholarship to do a Masters at the University of Chicago in Islamic History and Arabic, a course I could only dream about and did not believe such a prestigious university would offer a scholarship to an Australian, living in Cairo with a broken neck.

Miracles do happen however and my Cairo background was amazingly what Chicago wanted for its Masters. And so, in August 1980, after nearly four years in Cairo learning about the Middle East, I headed for Chicago to do something fantastic with very little money but with a scholarship to cover my fees.

In my four years in Cairo, without doctors or pills, I maintained my usual average two seizures per year.

Chicago represented another enormous leap culturally, socially and intellectually. I was not unfamiliar with the US because of growing up in a US-inspired Australia and travelling across the US a decade earlier, but coming from Cairo it was all very new and exciting. And UoC was an intellectual hothouse unlike anything I had ever experienced. Never underestimate anybody was the golden rule which I learnt there and adhere to still.

My initial pals, all of us living at International House (I-House) on 59th Street, were an eclectic bunch of super-bright people, generally a few years younger than myself, and it was easy to develop a friendship group at I-House and with the 15-20 in my particular programme. I learnt quickly that UoC was extremely tough and rigorous. I found the hour and a half Arabic class five mornings a week at 9am plus the same amount of homework extremely demanding. And that was just one of my four subjects. It was a learning feast but you had to work enormously hard to do and understand the reading. Nevertheless, it was a superb intellectual environment with amazing resources and attitude.

My main professor, Marvin Zonis, who offered me the scholarship, acted as my politics professor and mentor and I am pleased to say that over 30 years later today he writes for my magazine and I write occasionally for his political blog. He and fellow student Dan Brumberg, now a politics professor at Georgetown University in Washington, remain great friends and I am hugely grateful to Marvin for giving me the opportunity to go to Chicago.

Did Marvin, Dan and my pals at UoC know about my epilepsy? I did not mention it to Marvin at any time but my friends were well aware, especially Scotty, who was a medical student at UoC and a flat mate after I-House and very helpful when it came to medical issues.

While we all worked hard, we played hard too. The usual drill for my pals was to stop studying around 11pm and go down to the nearby pub for a few beers and return after midnight. Some friends, Gina Titunik in particular, would start studying again and go through to 4am or more. Gina was a former sergeant in the US Marines who had got a GI Scholarship to do a PhD on Max Weber; Gina, like many others, was amazing but a good drinker too.

Unlike others, I had to earn my living as well. My scholarship covered my fees only. So I set about finding some jobs and got lucky by somehow getting a National Insurance Number which was essential for any paid work. Besides running the basement sandwich bar in I-House, I was also employed by the Chicago Urban Skills Institute as an English language teacher and so I was able to pay my mandatory medical insurance and buy a few beers, not much more. I was in heaven, learning what I did not know in Cairo about the Middle East, loving the UoC environment and having great pals, Gina, Dot, Scotty, Dan Brumberg and many more.

For the Chicago Institute I started teaching recently arrived Romanian immigrants who knew no English and because of my experience at the British Council in Cairo in teaching English to first-timers I loved the experience and the Romanians, in a poor part of South Chicago, were great fun. Over the next year or two I had various jobs at the Institute, including teaching at the black Kennedy-King Junior College, where I was the only white, and at a black old people's home on 39th Street where I was employed as an entertainer on Wednesday afternoons. I became an expert Bingo caller and provider of Al Jolson songs and films from the 1930s and members loved being serenaded by their Aussie white honky, I loved it too.

On a musical note we greatly enjoyed going to the blues clubs on the South Side and actually seeing great names such as Buddy Guy, Junior Wells and Muddy Waters. At I-House a band, called O2, was playing at an event, I made sandwiches for them all, but little did I realise how important they would become.

I studied hard, drank hard and took the summer semester in 1982 while doing multiple jobs and having a ball. By December 1982 I was finishing my courses and my Masters and had one final Arabic exam to complete. I was not a great Arabic student but broadly acceptable. The problem was I had a seizure on the morning of my last Arabic exam undoubtedly due to stress. I did not make it to the exam, I was very upset. But my professor, who had seen me almost every day for the past 15 months, knew me well and knew what I could and could not do and fortunately she gave me a pass without me having to resit the exam. Even UoC had some understanding for my epilepsy and I graduated with my Masters later that month, a very happy boy.

I had achieved my Masters but what next? Luck followed me in Chicago and under the US system a foreign post-graduate could work for a year if the conditions were right. Marvin, amazingly noted a vacancy for a Country Risk Analyst for the Middle East at the city's largest bank, First Chicago.

Curiously, the fellow in the job was taking a year out and I turned out to be a well qualified substitute and so in January I started at First Chicago on a graduate salary of over $30,000, an absolute fortune for me at that time. And I could continue to live with friends in an apartment in Hyde Park near I-House, it was a dream situation although I had little knowledge of what a Country Risk Analyst did. Again, another comprehensive reeducation working in a flash bank in downtown Chicago as a Middle East expert with a salary. Wow.

1982 was another important year for me and my future. I was gradually gaining some traction and improving my lot despite the odd seizure. I was not on any medication but a medical student, Scotty Bohon, lived with us in Hyde Park and all seemed well.

First Chicago was indeed an education in a pre-Internet world in which I could not even call the Middle East because of the huge time difference. I sat in Chicago with few resources, if any, and was meant to pontificate on the Middle East, provide estimates on OPEC oil prices and be wise when there was only guesswork. I got used to Chicago's isolation from my Middle East and while my boss, Alan Stoga, had his doubts over me I was able to meet requirements.

My social life expanded and I had plenty of money for partying and Chicago was/is a magnificent place even if extremely cold at times. I had hitch hiked down to stay with good friends, the Rankins in North Carolina at Christmas 1982 and while very different than hitching in 1971 it was a rewarding experience but eventually replaced by flights.

As 1982 wore on it was absolutely clear I needed a new job and I was very keen to stay in the US, it was what I knew. But as is the case 35 years later in the UK, visas for foreigners were difficult and I was a foreigner and although Gina offered to marry me to keep me in the US, that was too much to ask. In the autumn I received a job offer from Houston, Texas and flew down to check it out.

The Houston folk were pleased to hire me and asked me immediately to go out and look for an apartment. But my health played against me. I had to admit that I did not have a driving licence due to my epilepsy and in an instant the job evaporated and I was sent back to Chicago empty handed. Houston is not possible without a car and so in surveying the US outlook, my prospects on all fronts looked bleak.

One gets lucky at times. I was so frustrated at my visa/health problems in the US I decided to make a direct call to the Middle East magazine I used at First Chicago and ask them directly for a job. The magazine, Middle East Economic Digest (MEED), was based in London and I called directly the Editor, Richard

Purves. As luck had it I got through to him directly from Chicago and I unashamedly put my case. I was desperate.

Curiously, as luck would have it, they were looking for someone with a finance/Middle East background but naturally they needed to know whether I could do the job. Unlike the US, the UK authorities at that time would go into bat for a foreigner they wanted, so a visa was not a particular obstacle in the UK. And again with luck there was a gap in MEED's Washington bureau and so they offered to test me out in Washington and if I passed muster I would be able to come across to the UK a few months later.

Although I was reluctant to leave friends in sweet home Chicago and the Rankins in North Carolina I had no choice, the US appeared not available to me. MEED was my big chance and I took it. So in late November I left First Chicago and headed to Washington where I could stay for a few months with old friend Haywood Rankin who had a house there as a US diplomat and so I was back in Middle East journalism in earnest. I had known Haywood since my early days in Cairo and he was well aware of my epilepsy exploits there and had helped with various visas to both the UK and the US.

Washington was another eye-opener for me. I was in the centre of global politics and as a Middle East journalist I felt the full force of politics in Washington, the influence of the lobbying groups and in particular the Israeli lobbying groups. At the time the deal for the Saudi AWACs surveillance planes was going through Congress and in my humble MEED office one felt the power of the Israeli lobbies keen to quash the AWACs deal. It passed, I learnt a lot and in the Press Building the Financial Times office was immediately next to MEED's. There I met Anatole Kaletsky, the FT's Washington bureau chief (now a columnist with The Times) ; I always read his columns and was amazed at his intelligence. I realised how hard it was to be good; Anatole was the gold standard, I was struggling at first but quickly used my experience to write some good copy that passed muster and in March I was heading for London.

Haywood Rankin was hugely helpful in my Washington stint, I absorbed all that the capital had to offer and loved it, the politics, the museums, the music and the Washington Redskins too. But I had done my time as correspondent and now I had to establish myself in my new head office in London. Again I was lucky, my good friend Martin Rose offered me his flat in Hungerford Road N7, about 100 yards from where we live today in Beacon Hill and other friends Heather and Celia Simpson allowed me to stay in Richmond with them when I arrived.

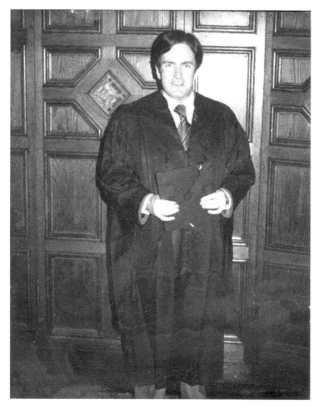

Chicago friends, (from left) Gina Titunik, Steve T., Mike, Tom Clay, in our flat in 1981

Graduating from University of Chicago with a Masters degree in Islamic History and Arabic in 1981.

IN HIGHBURY, LONDON

Arriving in London was definitely the start of a new phase of my life and 34 years later when writing this book I am still living in London not far away from where I started and less than a mile from the Arsenal Football Club stadium. While I have always lived within kicking distance of Arsenal a lot has changed for me since I arrived in 1983 although some may argue a lot has stayed the same.

I continue as a journalist and writer, I retain my good friends, especially Gail, who was my boss in 1977 and became my wife in 1987 and in 2017 we had our 30th anniversary in Bellagio on Lake Como where we had our honeymoon. Also Martin Rose, who I met on my first day at *The Egyptian Gazette* in 1977 and who was the best man at my wedding and is still a regular visitor at our house in Beacon Hill.

But one important change was the arrival of Liberty Rose Juliet Timewell, our daughter, in October 1988. She has been an amazing delight to us both from the start and now we visit her as a UK diplomat in Beijing, she the rising star and us the busy, retired doting parents.

Of course all this was in the future when I landed in London in early 1983 and began at Middle East Economic Digest (MEED). What I did know then, however, was I loved the journalism I was involved in, I was lucky to have this opportunity at MEED and I was keen to pursue it. Also MEED was willing, unlike firms in the US, to go in to bat for me to obtain the necessary visas and so I soon had my permanent residency in the UK which I still use decades later. For the first time in seven years I had no visa problems, I was a permanent resident at last.

At the magazine, which I knew well as a reader, I was welcomed in almost a family atmosphere and quickly slotted in to its weekly rhythms. The owner, Jonathan Wallace, my boss, Eddie O'Sullivan and my colleagues all became firm friends and much time was spent cavorting in the nearby pub, The Duke of York.

1983 was a year of consolidation and stability. Work was going well, I was loving Martin's flat in Hungerford Road and my health was under control. I had met an Egyptian doctor, Magdi Omar, and he became a close friend and my doctor too, and after a lapse of several years I was back on anti-epilepsy medication. In those early London years I still had seizures, averaging around two a year, but like my teenage years they were generally at home and in the early morning, and nothing to greatly worry about.

As I moved into the mid-1980s a new found fresh sense of stability came over me. I was travelling to new places, I was in a secure job which I loved, I was surrounded by a friendly and happy environment and with reasonable finances I even managed to buy a magnificent two-bedroom flat with a large garden in Highbury New Park. How good was this?

Although grand efforts to revive a relationship with an old Australian flame failed dismally in Paris, I could now think positively for once and the disasters in my past in Australia were well behind me.

Little did I know what new opportunities the MEED 1985 Christmas party would bring. As always we had a Christmas raffle and I was asked to select the winner; curiously I selected myself and despite cries of "rigged" I held firm and won a flight for two to anywhere in Europe. I knew this was my golden opportunity to ask Gail to Istanbul and I did it and so began our romance that still lasts today.

Gail was working in Milan for the British Council and I was slow and unsure how to make my play, the raffle provided the ready answer.

Istanbul got things started and I spent the rest of 1986 planning trips to Milan, visits to Bellagio along with work trips to Saudi Arabia and the Middle East. Christmas 1986 Gail and I spent with all the Rose family in their wonderful cottage in the Black Mountains village of Cymyoy. It was an amzing time in Wales but what followed was even more amazing.

In the new year we had driven north to Newcastle and coming back to London on the A46 out of Lincoln I somehow suggested to Gail driving her Mini that she should come to live with me in London but then I went to sleep. At the Rose's house in Hampstead, London, Jocelyn Rose spotted something in the air and after 40 minutes of prevarication and fumbling we announced our engagement. Slow Steve eventually did it.

While there was little of medical significance happening in these years there was plenty happening socially and at work. It was all very positive and although I had seizures, they did not interrupt my life. My Egyptian friend and doctor, Magdi Omar, helped with medication and gave me confidence on the epilepsy front. All was working well.

Gail and I planned our 1987 wedding for the 15th August, on the day of the Assumption, in Catholic terms, and amidst all this a couple of friends from MEED, Eddie O'Sullivan and Dave Hawley, and myself made an ambitious bid to buy our magazine with the help of investment banker friend, George Kanaan. We were outbid with an offer of £2.6million but while my entrepreneurial spirit was crushed somewhat the wedding went ahead in fine style in our back garden at Highbury New Park with over 120 in attendance on a marvellous summer day with Martin as best man. I was a lucky boy indeed. Back in Cairo days I thought Gail was absolutely terrific but I never believed it would be possible to marry her. As has happened often in my curious life, amazing things can happen, all things are possible as they say.

Over ten years after leaving Australia with my tail between my legs I was slowly at last getting my act together - I was married to a tremendous person who knew me warts and all, I had a career and also a lovely flat. But 1988 brought me something extra – wonderful little Liberty on 13 October.

But before Liberty something significant happened in August. My sister Julie called to say that her husband, Tom Ericksen (52), had died. Julie was left with six children under 16, no money, no title to her house and thus a mountainous road to climb. I sat in the newsroom and felt a great burden had been taken off me, I felt massively relieved. Tom had been the source of many of my problems for years but now he was gone. Julie, however, needed a lot of help and although I went out to Australia to do what I could, there was little of substance I could do. Julie had to battle on, get the kids through school and survive which she has done remarkably well.

Back in London, after missing a Michael Jackson concert and being arrested as a diamond-watch smuggler at Gatwick bringing back a watch Julie wanted me to sell at Garrards, the jeweller (a very long story), I waited for the arrival of Gail's bump. They were stressful times but we all came through it and when beautiful, blond Liberty appeared we decided, with Gail's mother's help, that the best thing we could do was take Liberty to Australia for a family Christmas. A new young life partially compensating for the loss of Julie's husband.

Liberty was a magnificent baby, and was a great tonic for her Aussie cousins. And I will always remember Granny Nora sitting on the surf beach at Portsea at age 78, the first time she had ever set foot on a surf beach anywhere.

Babies grow quickly and it wasn't long into 1989 when we were beginning to outgrow Highbury New Park and we began to look further afield. It was also tough times at MEED and its more expensive finance editor had to be let go. Despite the stress, I remained medically sound and, again with luck, found a new job as Editor of Arab Banker, the magazine of the Arab Bankers Association, and Gail found a job at South Bank University to improve the family finances. We were fortunate.

Amongst all this we found a lovely, modern three-bedroom house in Elfort Road adjacent to Arsenal's old Highbury stadium and Gail and I thought we were set. Liberty was doing well, we had jobs, although mine was rather poorly paid, and Elfort Road was great. What more could we want?

Gail and Steve T. in the 1980s

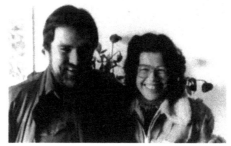

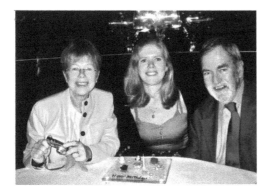

Gail, Liberty and Steve at Pied à Terre restaurant in Charlotte Street (picture taken by Tom) on Liberty's 20th birthday.

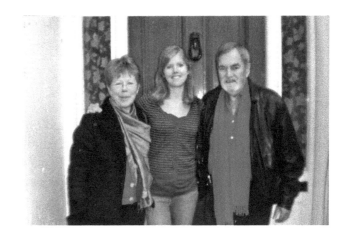

*Gail, Liberty and Steve
at Beacon Hill.*

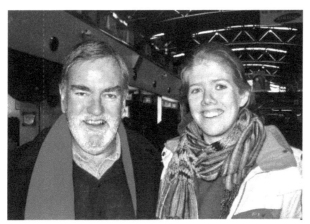

Steve and Liberty in Beijing.

29 BEACON HILL

The early 1990s were somewhat benign with some key exceptions. Liberty was a delight, expanding her abilities thanks to her Mum and being everything a young toddler could ever want to be. Gail was doing well at London South Bank University, although with the usual staff clashes, and I managed to move from Arab Banker to The Banker, part of the Financial Times, in 1990. An old friend from MEED, Gavin Shreeve, had been appointed Editor of The Banker in around 1988 and he needed a Middle East specialist and I jumped at the opportunity and the rise in salary too.

So the early 1990s saw a glowing Liberty, her Mum and Dad doing well in their jobs and all happily ensconced in Elfort Road. My health faded from the picture at that time; while I kept detailed records of my seizures from 1991, I was pleased to report that between 1991-95 I only had two seizures, one in the summer of 1991 at Elfort Road and one in the summer of 1995 in the early morning in Tallin, Estonia on a business trip. This benign period was not to last with 11 seizures between 1996-2000 (see Table) and many more after that.

Epilepsy has many aspects and over a number of decades it is important to appreciate that it can even have some humorous aspects as well. One family legend dates back to a seizure in the summer of 1991 at Elfort Road. Gail recalls a huge crashing sound upstairs in our bedroom one Sunday morning. Oblivious to the great sounds myself, Gail came up to find that I had seemingly rugby tackled our bed from a standing position and completely destroyed the bed.

The bed was in pieces sprawled across the room and I was spread-eagled across it with massive damage to my face and head. I was obviously completely out of it but I do remember waking up with incredible dark bruising to my face and upper body. The bed was history and we had to laugh. You could not plan to do such a thing but somehow I managed to rugby tackle and destroy our bed during this seizure. Fortunately, not all seizures have those results and despite the damage to my face the bruising disappeared over night and I went off to work on the Monday and we needed a new bed.

The 'rugby tackle' seizure was perhaps the most amusing of many strange events, the motor cycle seizure in Cairo being the most dramatic and most destructive, but at least I was wearing a helmet, if I did not have one I would not be writing this. A few months after this I was shown my wrecked helmet, it was severely damaged, I was a very lucky boy as I have said often in this text.

The early 1990s were a particularly good time but the somewhat relative calm was however disturbed when Gail's Mum, Granny Nora, suggested to Gail she would like to come and live with us. We knew that Elfort Road was good for three people but not for four, so we needed to find a new house with a proper space for Granny. Did we have the funds for all this? Not really, but with a lot of fussing around, help and family politics we moved into an amazing six-bedroom house with a perfect granny flat in Beacon Hill in August 1993. While we could have been gazumped by a group of nuns who also wanted it, the owner chose our family and we bought this mansion for £235,000, a tenth of its value nearly 25 years later. Again we were lucky and Granny was pleased too.

29 Beacon Hill provided the foundation for our years ahead. Many family members, including nieces Sally and Mari Ericksen and nephew Tom Ericksen along with many others, stayed with us over the years, we had six bedrooms plus Granny's flat, so no shortage of space and a back garden perfect for big barbies and there were and are still plenty of those. Liberty had her 21st birthday at Beacon Hill in 2009 with over 80 in attendance, a grand affair.

The 1990s were a consolidation period for Gail and I after some turbulent times. There were crises of course, like all young or relatively young parents bringing up Liberty, paying the mortgage and the beginning of school fees kept us busy. Gail was progressing at South Bank University and in 1992 my friend Gavin decided to leave The Banker for better things and all of a sudden I was made Editor. I had my dream job but seriously wondered whether it was all possible. The FT thought they would give me a try and it all happened.

I remember asking Gavin, somewhat naively: "How do you know how you are going?" He replied: "If you are still there after three years you are doing fine." Well in 2017, after 25 years, I am still on the masthead as Editor Emeritus, so I must have been doing something right.

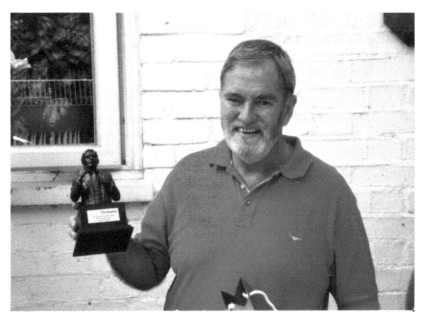

Steve with his own Bracken banking award in his own backyard.

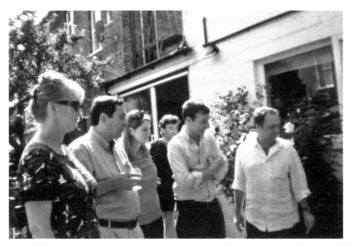

Some of The Banker crew at the annual Banker barbie at Beacon Hill.

I struggled with being Editor in the early days but I concentrated on continuing to pursue my interests in the Middle East and travel as much as I could to new areas as well. The Banker was a truly global magazine and I had to be credible in all areas of the world not just my old stomping grounds.

As can be seen by my rough travel chart of the 1990s (compiled by analysis of passports at that time) my adventures broadened out from the Middle East in the 1980s to many countries in Asia, including China and Japan, as well as central and eastern Europe

and central Asia, including, Kazakhstan, Russia, Hungary and the Czech Republic. I expanded my own personal brief to well beyond the Middle East and covered central Europe and central Asia. I fully believed I had the best job in the world and as the Soviet Empire declined all these new states emerged and needed to be covered. It was the perfect opportunity to bring some of these states and their banks to world attention and I was keen to take advantage of these opportunities for the magazine.

While the opportunities were there and I attempted to do my best I was travelling a lot and my home life suffered. I clearly was not home as much as I should have been and this put increased pressures on Gail and Liberty. It also put increased pressures on myself and it is perhaps no surprise that between 1996-2000 I had 11 seizures but again I was fortunate that most of these were in the morning at home and did not do me any great damage. While I did have a minor seizure with old friends in southern France in 2005, it again passed without trace and I was particularly fortunate that while this period did provide considerably more travel and stress in running the magazine it did not produce significantly adverse outcomes. My index of seizures from 1991 onwards helps explain what was going on in my life from a health perspective.

The 1990s involved not only considerable work travel abroad but as a family we also travelled a number of times to Australia, including an amazing visit to the Great Barrier Reef in glorious Queensland during the 1996 Olympics in Atlanta. It was truly memorable to go swimming in the coral islands off Port Douglas, we remember the trip with great affection. We were fortunate to keep in touch with our many relatives in and around Melbourne and some in Sydney too and Liberty certainly got to know her cousins better and get a feel for Australia. She has dual citizenship, UK and Australian, I remain with just my Aussie passport.

The 21st century brought more travel and an exciting time for The Banker with many global financial developments and changes in the global economy. Just as I had done in the 1990s I attended all the big global meetings such as the annual meetings of the IMF/World Bank in Washington or wherever. The magazine was expanding and all the Timewells, including Liberty, were performing well and exceeding expectations.

But the new decade also brought signs of considerable wear and tear. While I was travelling more and developing more new areas, such as The Banker Global Banking Awards in 2000, I was now 50 and the strain was beginning to show. Between 2001-2005 I had nine seizures, again nothing too dramatic except a seizure in a hotel in Tehran just before a special government-arranged trip to the holy city of Qom for Friday prayers. I managed to stay broadly conscious during the visit; on these rather important occasions I was going to keep up appearances no matter how badly I felt.

As the decade wore on the stress continued to show and between 2006-2008 when the global financial crisis emerged I had 17 seizures in that three year period. My annual average number of seizures or 'turns' went up dramatically, I was under more stress and it showed.

While I obviously was not responsible for the global financial crisis, I believed that as Editor-in-Chief I should be able to understand what was going on and to articulate it for our readers. The truth was I didn't understand what was happening and all this confusion added to my stress levels. As can be seen in the diary of my seizures there was a lot happening in the second half of 2008, such as visits to Greece, Awards judging, the 2nd Islamic Summit plus the impact

of the nightsweats I was experiencing nightly led to nine seizures in 2008, my worst score so far. The global financial markets were in uproar, I, not surprisingly, had no answer, I was stressed and the seizures kept coming.

At work there was a realisation that I was not in good shape. I, of course, did not want to admit it. I was in denial. In late November it was felt that I should take a break and reluctantly I agreed to take a few weeks off; my last day was 26th November. I did not really accept that I had a problem but my body was telling me otherwise. Gail and others coaxed me into submission.

So 2008 ended, Lehman Brothers had gone down in September and the financial crisis of that year was seen by many economists to have been the worst financial crisis since the Great Depression of the 1930s.

There were massive bailouts to prevent the collapse of the world's financial system but what followed was a global economic downturn and the so-called Great Recession. It was not a pretty picture.

Did the world's financial gurus know what was going on? Definitely not, but they muddled through, and people like myself just had to stay calm and rest. I began to realise slowly that I had a problem, I accepted the issues facing me and the discussion of retirement emerged. I was 58 at the end of 2008, I did not think I was past it but my record of nine seizures in the year told a different story.

Something had to change. The seizures had seriously messed me about. I was not well and needed to get better and the Financial Times and Pearson, my employers, were incredibly good in looking after me. I was my worst enemy at times but in 2009 my perspectives began to change and less stress (from being off work) and significantly more sleep, getting at least nine hours rather than seven, saw my health improve.

Although it was tough I began to accept that I had to change and in April I accepted my formal retirement. The FT was exceptionally generous to me and boosted my retirement age from 58 to the statutory 62 and so again I was very fortunate in terms of my pension and payouts. I had been there since 1990 and The Banker had progressed well under me and my successor Brian Caplen who I had hired.

Again I was very lucky but while I had formally retired that was not the end of the line for me and The Banker. I had to change and adapt and 2009 was a transformational year not only for the world economy but also for me. Less stress and more sleep put me back on course and it was no accident that I had no seizures at all in 2009 after nine the previous year.

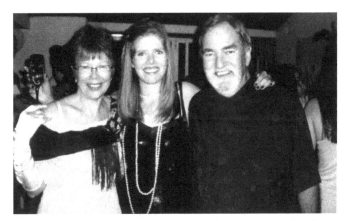

Liberty's 21st birthday party at Beacon Hill in October 2009 (Gail, Liberty and Steve T.)

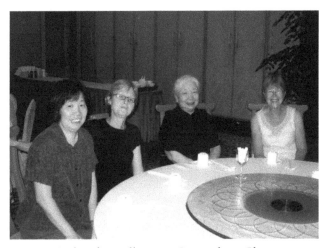

Gail and ex colleagues, Guangzhou, China.
Li Hai Li, Sue Maingay, Lao Li and Gail in 2009.

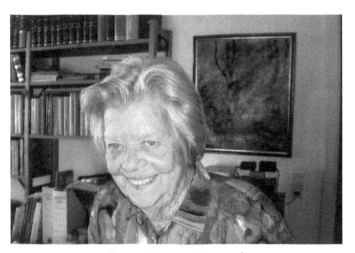

Granny Bente in Denmark.

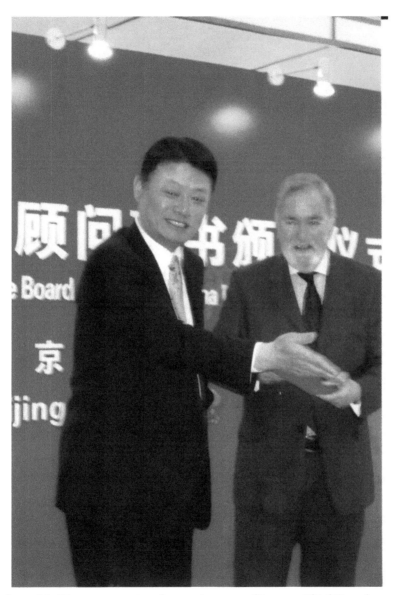

President of Minsheng, Mr Hong announcing the appointment of Steve as Chief Consultant on May 9th 2011

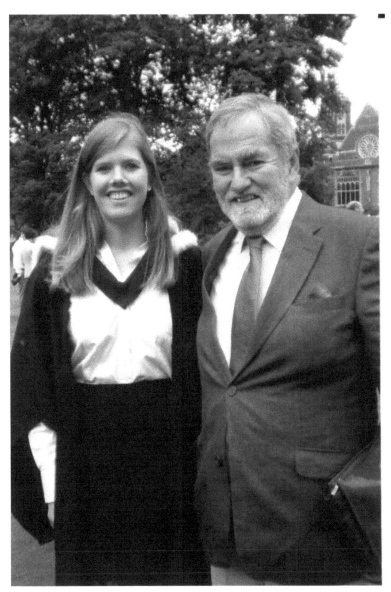

Liberty and Steve on Liberty's Graduation Day in Cambridge in 2012.

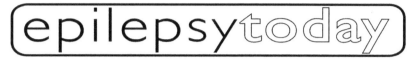

Epilepsy Today is the magazine of *Epilepsy Action*.

THE MAN WITH THE MEMOIRS: MY FIRST SEIZURE

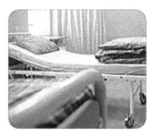

Stephen Timewell continues to ruminate on his life with epilepsy. In his latest column instalment, he recalls a confusing event that will be familiar to many readers: his very first seizure.

I was 13 and in my 9th year of school and as usual after breakfast I walked down to the bus stop nearby to go to school on the other side of Melbourne. I didn't get there. From being at the bus stop I was suddenly somewhere else. I seemed to be in the clouds but as things became clearer the clouds were plain clear curtains and I was in a room. I initially thought I was in heaven and I must have died. I thought heaven a strange place but as the minutes passed I came down to earth and realised I was in some kind of hospital room. I looked through the curtains and saw a familiar road outside, New Street. I slowly took on board I was in a private hospital I knew well on the corner of New Street and Normanby Street, about 400 yards from home and the bus stop.

I was completely flummoxed. I knew where I was but how did I get there, what had happened? I started to realise too that my mouth was damaged and painful and I seemed to have lost a tooth. From thoughts of being in heaven I was feeling rather fuzzy and alarmed at where I was and why. I eventually composed myself in this fuzziness and yelled out.

Someone came and my new reality struck. I was in the private hospital with St Andrew's Church opposite, I was not in heaven but in rather bad shape. No one could tell me what had happened and I was in a confused and semi-conscious state. Writing this 50 years later I can still remember clearly the puzzled state I was in. And then somehow my parents arrived and carried me off home to bed and a lot of sleep.

Dad was very upset and I still didn't know what happened. But in the following days I heard the words epilepsy, fit, seizure and I realised something was seriously wrong but I didn't have a clear understanding of what went wrong at the bus stop and, curiously, 50 years later I am not that much better informed.

In my younger days Dad used to take me to a paediatrician, Dr Sinn, as I was believed to be highly strung. I didn't understand what this meant but I took the pills I was prescribed which was then known as dilantin (today known as phenytoin which I still take today). As I got older I moved away from Dr Sinn to Dad's specialist Dr Sewell, who began to look after me and clearly the bus stop seizure led to my visits to Dr Sewell who Dad had used for many years.

My first bus stop seizure was unfortunately followed by a number of other seizures in the following months. Most of these, as I remember, were at home in the morning before school. This led to Dad becoming increasingly upset and deciding to drive me to school every morning. This worked well because some school friends nearby came too and their parents helped in the school run.

For me, the seizures did not cause much damage to me physically and I went to school and carried on as usual. I knew there was a stigma attached to epilepsy but it was not mentioned at school and I did not let it affect me and I was fortunate not to have any seizures at school. I was concerned but the half dozen grand mal seizures I had in that first year did not bother me greatly and I just got on with school and everything else.

But as the seizures continued a disturbed Dad took me to Dr Sewell more often and I remember one meeting with the doctor very, very clearly. In trying to explain what these grand mal seizures meant Dr Sewell said very clearly that I could not expect to finish school, I could not expect to go to university and that I could not expect to do a lot of things. I had already been told that I could not drive a car or related things but I was only 13 and a good way away from my licence anyway. But Dr Sewell saying I might not finish school and not go to university really upset me and certainly beefed up my determination to prove him wrong and do so.

Why the doctor gave me this hard message is still a mystery to me. In hindsight it did not seem a way to lift my spirits and I still find it difficult to understand why he would give such a negative prognosis unless he wanted somehow to spur me on which I don't think was his purpose. Again in hindsight I don't think it was one of his better judgments but whether intended or not it certainly spurred me on to prove that I certainly could finish school and go to university regardless of whether I had epilepsy or however many fits I had.

When I was 14 Dad had the idea to try a chiropractor to see if he could 'straighten my spine' and reduce the number of fits I was having. For a year Dad took me twice a week to this chiropractor who seemingly made my spine look straighter and there was a corresponding reduction in the number of fits but it is hard to say the two events were related. I kept having fits and I became even more determined to do well at school and I did.

My knowledge of epilepsy was weak then and remains so today 50 years later as research has improved but still leaving a lot of imponderables. At 16, however, I finished school, quite young for my age and against the odds I got into my first choice and entered Monash University when I was 17 to study economics. I still had fits and I still took my pills but I had made it to university despite what Dr Sewell had said and I was very pleased to prove him wrong.

And by the time I was 20 I had the degree and did not let epilepsy put a damper on any of my aspirations.

And now, 50 years after my first fit, I still have regular tonic-clonic or grand mal seizures and I still take my pills (phenytoin) but I have a Masters degree from the University of Chicago, have had a very successful career in journalism and a very happy family life. I must add with no thanks to Dr Sewell.

THE MAN WITH THE MEMOIRS:
HOW A SEIZURE ALMOST LED TO
AN INTERNATIONAL INCIDENT

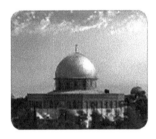

16 April, 2014

Stephen Timewell continues to recount an eventful life with epilepsy. In this tale, he recollects a key moment in Middle Eastern history – and how it was almost put at risk by a very poorly timed seizure

Politics and seizures do not tend to go together. But towards the end of 1977 some cataclysmic global political events had some major ramifications which included what can only be described as a 'politically-induced seizure' and its potentially bizarre political consequences.

This curious story dates back to early November 1977 when President Anwar Sadat of Egypt agreed to become the first Arab leader ever to visit the state of Israel. Breaking this political logjam was a massive breakthrough and as I was a journalist with the Cairo-based government-owned daily newspaper, The Egyptian Gazette, there was a lot to discuss and a lot to be done with this momentous occasion.

My Egyptian Editor believed that the Gazette should be represented at this historic event and I was selected to go in the advance press plane to be there at Ben Gurion Airport in Israel when President Sadat arrived. To say I was excited to go was a complete understatement as Egyptians could hardly believe Sadat was going to meet the Israelis in Israel and Sadat's move had turned the global political world, let alone the Middle East, completely upside down.

History was being made and even I, as an Australian- born Egyptian journalist, was making history, taking the first commercial flight ever from Egypt to Israel. It was a unique political occasion, a completely unprecedented event and over 35 years later I can still remember the tension and excitement as the press corps stood behind the Israeli dignitaries at the airport as the plane carrying Sadat approached.

It was so bizarre that many thought that rather than Sadat the plane would contain a group of armed militias who would mow down the Israelis and the press standing behind. This did not happen fortunately. Sadat met Israeli Prime Minister Menachem Begin and the start of the peace process was begun. Sadat delivered his speech to the Israeli Knesset on 20 November 1977 and I made the first telephone call (from Israel to Egypt) to report back to our Cairo office (the Israeli operator was more excited than me).

It was thrilling to be a part of this piece of history and the atmosphere was surreal. Could this really be the start of a peace process? There was a huge amount of optimism and excitement in the air and as an English-speaking Egyptian journalist I was feted by Israeli and foreign journalists alike. A Canadian journalist even wrote a special feature about me, entitled "Blue-eyed Arab".

The Israelis wanted to show some of the visiting Egyptians some parts of Israel and a visit was planned to the Dead Sea, not that far from Jerusalem. This is where an unlikely turn of events took place and demonstrated the unlikely consequences of an unexpected epileptic seizure.

There was no shortage of excitement while I was in Israel and the trip to the Dead Sea was perhaps a bit of excitement too far. The result was I had a seizure somewhere at the Dead Sea and the Israeli officials were suddenly aware that they were in the midst of a serious cross-border international incident. For them I was an Egyptian, until two days ago their mortal enemy, and given the success of the Sadat-Begin visit so far they were very keen that nothing go wrong. Having an Egyptian in a bad state of health was not good and as in most such cases the officials were not sure what was wrong and whether a crisis could be avoided.

And so when I recovered some consciousness in hospital I could see a bevy of concerned faces surrounding me, anxiously trying to figure out my condition and whether fragile Egyptian-Israeli relations were in further jeopardy.

Regaining some consciousness I was able to explain my medical condition to the doctors and the Israeli foreign ministry personnel who had gathered around me. The last thing they wanted was news that an Egyptian had died in an Israeli hospital at this specific time. But fortunately their worst fears were easily allayed. I had just had an ordinary epileptic seizure, I would recover readily and there was no political fallout to be concerned about.

I was only 26 at the time, I recovered relatively quickly and I could see the relief lifting away from these officials as I slowly came back to normal. And so the Sadat visit continued, we all returned to Cairo without further incident and decades later peace between Egypt and Israel remains prickly at best, but my seizure on that first visit fortunately did not add to the problems.

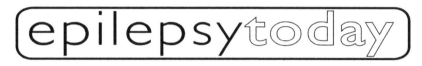

THE MAN WITH THE MEMOIRS:
FROM A SEIZURE TO A SCHOLARSHIP

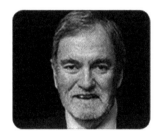

6 November, 2013

Our new regular columnist, Stephen Timewell, recalls an event in the late 70s – a terrible motorcycle accident that should have spelled the end of his life… but strangely, took it in a new direction entirely

Having seizures can be frustrating and sometimes depressing. There is no easy way to ignore them or their effects. Still, a positive approach is important – out of all bad comes some good. It is possible to construct something meaningful out of the darkest of moments.

The following tale is curiously true – and they do say that truth is stranger than fiction. Back in the 70s I was in my twenties. I found myself working in Cairo (Egypt) enjoying a profession I'd only just discovered: teaching.

I was teaching English in an Egyptian private secondary school and found I liked it a great deal. Unfortunately, I also found that I needed to supplement my meagre income. This took me into journalism at the local English language newspaper, *The Egyptian Gazette* (founded in 1880).

Both these Egyptian salaries did not amount to much. Fortunately, the desire of the British Council (BC) to establish a Teaching Centre soon created a huge opportunity for people like myself (even despite my Australian accent). The BC needed teachers and paid enormously well by my standards at the time in 1977.

Two friends and I appeared before a delightful London- appointed teacher (our boss) called Gail. We were promptly hired. Gail had a motorbike. It wasn't long before my friend Martin and I also had motorbikes – and the three of us became the Hell's Angels of Cairo! (Although I felt rather underpowered on my orange Czech Jawa 175cc bike.)

I had epilepsy and was still having seizures – so why did I decide to ride a motorbike? I decided that the Cairo traffic was so dreadfully slow that the only person I could kill was myself. The bike would certainly help me getting to work at school and the Teaching Centre.

At 26, getting the motorbike licence did not represent a problem. There were no questions relevant to my epilepsy. There I was – happily riding to school, the BC, out to the Pyramids at full moon… and enjoying driving for the first time in my life.

Was I stupid? Yes, but in the Cairo of 1977, I decided to ride my luck and hope for the best. Amazing things were happening at the time. President Sadat decided he did not want more Egyptians to die fighting Israel and opted to go to Israel himself. As an Egyptian journalist I was assigned to go with him, amazingly enough. It was, and still is, the most politically important trip of my life. All things were possible – but they were about to change for me.

Soon after arriving back from Israel, my family in Melbourne informed me – for their various reasons – that they wanted me to move to Syria immediately. The full reasons of why they wanted me to go to Syria is a long, complex story, suffice to say I was devastated and upset and clearly did not want to go, but could see no alternative. That night I sought solace with my friend in drinking many, *many* beers. It was a heavy night and certainly I paid for it in the morning when I got up for school.

It was a 10km ride on my Jawa to school in the Cairo suburb of Maadi. I did not make it. Outside Cairo's main teaching hospital – Kasr El-Aini – I had a seizure on the Jawa and crashed head first into a tree. Remarkably, unlike most Egyptians, I wore a helmet – which probably saved my life… but over two days later, I woke up in the Kasr Al-Aini hospital with a broken neck. My driving days were ended forever.

I was in bad shape, but alive. Friends at *The Egyptian Gazette* and my boss, Gail, were surprised by my absence. They started looking for me and found me in the ward for broken necks. They tried to shield me when the patient next to me, Mohammed, stopped breathing – but I knew it was all pretty grim. For the moment, I was lucky to be alive and not paralysed.

Despite Kasr Al-Aini being a teaching hospital, nursing is not well developed in Egypt. Gail was shocked when so- called nurses lumbered me onto beds for X-rays. I was lucky to survive the nursing treatment. Tariq – a friend of Martin's – was a medical professor. He warned me that I would die in that ward unless he got me out. Tariq took me to his home so I would not die in hospital.

I survived the following weeks at Tariq's. I didn't go to Syria and my family remained out of touch. My broken neck mended in the wrong position, but I could move my head (with some difficulty) and I was still alive. The physiotherapy I'd been recommended should have killed me, but somehow it didn't. Over the course of 1978, I slowly returned to my old life, somewhat the worse for wear.

At school, the chance came about to lead a group of 16 girls and boys to England and Scotland in the summer of 1978. This gave me an opportunity to also see these places – and also take my X-rays to specialists in Edinburgh. So it happened and with great success.

In Edinburgh my consultant, Mr Harris, informed me delicately that if I'd been British he would not let me leave his room. I wasn't British. So we struck a deal for an operation on my neck for £2,000 when I had the money. He added somewhat humorously: "Be careful at the lights." He meant that if I stopped sharply my neck was in serious danger. So, back I went to Cairo to somehow save up £2,000 for a dangerous operation that I may not live to see.

I was still having tonic-clonic seizures and my neck was still very fragile. Nevertheless, I saved the money somehow. In summer 1979, I arrived in Edinburgh to have my neck re- broken – with a good chance I would not survive. I knew I had to do it and that what would be would be.

When I did wake up after the operation I was surprised that they had to take a piece of bone out of my bottom to add to the metal they installed in my neck. Many times in my life I might have had my head in my ass. I think this was the first time I'd actually had my ass in my head. Still, I was alive.

The operation was finally over… But foolishly I had not even thought about recovery and what I would do when I got out of hospital. Fortunately, a Scottish girl – Katie, a friend of good pal Charles Richards in Cairo, came to my rescue. Katie offered to take me into her apartment – and became my true guardian angel.

While recovering at Katie's, I was reading *The Guardian* when I noticed an advertisement from the University of Chicago. The university was running a master's degree in Islamic History and Arabic. It sounded perfect for me, but I explained my fears to Katie. Would the University of Chicago ever give a scholarship to an Australian with a broken neck living in Cairo? I dismissed the idea completely,

but Katie insisted that since I was doing nothing I should apply. I reluctantly agreed. I sent off an application to a Prof Marvin Zonis, outlining my background in the Middle East and work at *The Egyptian Gazette*.

To my absolute astonishment, Marvin wanted someone with genuine experience in the Middle East to add to the master's programme. My CV fitted the bill. To my shock he *did* offer a scholarship to an Australian with a broken neck living in Cairo!

My career took off after gaining the master's degree in Islamic History and Arabic. It led to various successes in financial journalism – all this after breaking my neck having a seizure on a motorbike in Cairo and breaking my neck. It was a strange way to end up at the University of Chicago, but that was the starting point. As dark as some of those days were after the accident, somehow it all turned out for the good.

Also Gail, Martin and Marvin continue to play important roles in my life over 30 years later. Gail is now my wife. Martin continues to be my friend. Marvin is a valued mentor, someone I have worked with for all this time. So it really is important to continue to believe that out of all bad comes some good.

Stephen Timewell is Editor Emeritus of The Banker magazine, the global banking magazine of the Financial Times Group

stephen.timewell@ft.com

epilepsytoday

THE MAN WITH THE MEMOIRS: DON'T LET SEIZURES STOP YOU FLYING

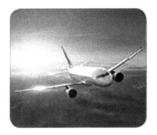

26 April, 2014

Stephen Timewell continues his column, remembering moments of his life with epilepsy. Here, he tries to puzzle out what triggered several.

For those who have seizures there are many issues and possible dangers. Falling over, damaging yourself, biting your tongue are just some problematic issues which can be upsetting, unsettling and deeply disturbing both to the epileptic and those around him or her. But in 2008, after 45 years of fits, I added a new dimension to my epilepsy record, having seizures on planes.

Having travelled the world continuously for work and pleasure since my early 20s, generally on my own, I was flying back from Dubai to London on an overnight flight after a four-day business trip in September 2008, when, I am told, I had what was called an average fit at 5.30am Wednesday morning. I, as usual, had no warning that a seizure was coming but landing in London even in my semi- conscious state I was well aware of the pandemonium I had caused. When I awoke there were lots of people fussing around me,

I was very embarrassed and I struggled to say anything. Fortunately, someone on the plane had seen this all before and understood what was going on and I believe calmed everybody down.

I was annoyed I had caused all this fuss and could not really say or do anything about it. Why did it happen? I had had another overnight flight on the way to Dubai, a busy schedule of interviews and meetings and a typically stressful time. All this could be seen as conducive to a seizure especially with broken sleep patterns and overnight flights. But this was my normal routine as an international financial journalist so why I should have had a seizure then I really don't know. I had taken my pills.

At Heathrow I was greeted by paramedics and some strange looks by surrounding passengers. But with some help, a wheelchair and some confusion on my part I collected my bag and was bundled into a taxi for home in north London. Once home I slept the rest of Wednesday and stayed very quiet Thursday.

Later that month I had another early morning fit after a stressful week in Greece but this time I was home in bed. My busy schedule continued and I had a total of nine seizures in 2008 (only one in a plane), something had to change.

2009 was a different year, my work programme slowed considerably, I officially retired (on the grounds of ill health) and I increased my sleep from seven to nine hours a night. Perhaps, not surprisingly, I was fortunate to have no seizures at all in 2009 and that seemed an improvement.

But 2010 brought other changes and significantly more fits, both in planes and elsewhere. On February 19th , after a few weeks seeing relatives in Australia I was heading back alone to London taking the long flight from Melbourne to Shanghai. Nine hours in I woke up surrounded by attendants having badly bitten my tongue and feeling rather confused. This time the plane experience was much worse than before but with my seat belt on I did not severely inconvenience other passengers. At Shanghai I had to manage to get my luggage and then catch a domestic flight to Beijing. This was one of the most difficult things I have ever done. I had a wheelchair but I was genuinely flying blind and barely conscious. It was nasty.

All I remember is that it was excruciating and a massive struggle to get on that domestic flight. Somehow I made it to the flight and as time passed I slowly felt a little better before the next challenge of getting to a hotel in Beijing. Again somehow in a complete mental fog I made it to a hotel and could collapse before flying back to London the next day. Why the fit on the flight to Shanghai? As with most of my epilepsy history direct factors behind the fits are difficult to fathom, there are indicators but no clear signs.

And so on a 22 April 2010 daytime flight to Riyadh from London I had a mild fit five hours into a seven hour flight. Although my mouth was badly damaged I managed to get off the plane unassisted, get to the hotel and perform my meetings reasonably well the next day. But two fits on two flights in two months was not good and again no credible reason could be found.

While I had three fits on three flights in this 2008-2010 period I have had no fits on planes in the almost four years since the flight to Riyadh. Despite a lot of plane travel there has been nothing since then although the number of total seizures hit 10 in 2010 and then dropped to four in both 2011 and 2012 and six in 2013.

What conclusions should one draw from all this? One could say I should lead a less stressful life, work less and not travel so much. Would this stop me having fits on planes? I am not sure. There seems to be no reliable correlation between work, stress, travel and fits on flights. I think to stop flying in order to avoid some fuss in planes and some definite inconvenience at airports is not the way to approach the issue. In my view it is necessary to just accept the seemingly random nature of these episodes and get on and enjoy the benefits that travel can bring.

Yes it is upsetting for other passengers and staff to have people like me having seizures on planes. I regret this. But epilepsy is just a medical condition, it is not the mythical, demonic condition that some seem to believe. The more epilepsy is understood the better it is for everyone. My only advice is don't let epilepsy stop you flying or doing anything for that matter, but as an assistance to fellow travellers it is always good to fasten your seat belt.

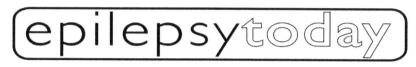

THE MAN WITH THE MEMOIRS: TELLING IS BETTER THAN NOT TELLING

Deciding when and how to tell young children about epilepsy in the family is often difficult and problematic, but not addressing the issue can cause problems too. The old adage 'damned if you do, damned if you don't' readily comes to mind. But a situation that arose when my daughter Liberty was aged seven, back in the early 1990s, clarified the issue for me.

While my wife and mother-in-law, who lived with us, were well aware of my epilepsy, we had not discussed it with Liberty. We were encouraged by the fact that in the period between 1992 and 1995, I had had no seizures; my last seizure was in the summer of 1991.

Out of sight, out of mind. The absence of seizures meant we neither thought nor talked about my epilepsy, which proved extremely unwise. Liberty was three when I had had the last seizure, and, at that point, we hadn't discussed my epilepsy with her. Then there was the three-year gap. In April 1996 my wife was away overseas on business and our au pair had the previous evening elected to stay with her boyfriend. Although she came back that morning, it was not early enough.

Early in the morning of 18 April, I had one of my normal tonic-clonic seizures. My daughter told me later that she had just come into the room and was watching me put my tie on when suddenly I keeled over backwards, wedged my head between the dressing table and the wall and then started convulsing with the usual big noise.

She was shocked to see this happen and apparently at the time thought I was dying. She had no idea what was going on and was hugely upset seeing her dad in such a state, mum abroad and not knowing what to do. Very luckily, her grandma was asleep in her flat downstairs. My daughter rushed downstairs to get her and with granny's help they got me back into bed and avoided calling an ambulance. The initial drama passed.

But for Liberty, what had happened to her father? I was unconscious and remained so for a number of hours before having a long sleep. Granny did her best to explain what had happened and I eventually recovered and could give some explanation myself. But the damage had been done. Liberty had to face this unfortunate drama completely unaware and not understanding what was happening.

She coped with all this, she had no option, but my wife and I regretted that she had not been better prepared and she had not better understood her father's condition. For most people, young or old, a tonic-clonic seizure represents quite a shock when first seen.

Although it is dramatic and possibly dangerous, it is generally not as bad as it first appears. Helping people of all ages understand seizures is very important in helping them better understand and deal with epilepsy. This is why I thoroughly recommend that young family members be made familiar with the meaning of someone in the family having a seizure. This will help them to learn what can be done during a seizure to make the person more comfortable and not endanger themselves.

Unfortunately, Liberty had to learn the hard way what a seizure meant. It would have been much better if her parents had given her more warning and better understanding of the reality of epilepsy. It is much better to be told in advance than to suffer the very strange experience of watching a tonic-clonic seizure and not understanding what is happening.

THE MAN WITH THE MEMOIRS:
HOW 72 SEIZURES BECAME A WORK OF ART

Having seizures is one thing but having an art exhibition based around a series of seizures is quite something else. Nevertheless, strange things emerge from odd places and to see a huge exhibition of my fits over a 20-year period in vivid colour in a 17-metre long landscape was clearly beyond my wildest imagination. If I had not witnessed hundreds of people trying to make sense of the *Timewell Timeline* I would not have believed it, but this did happen in the Beyond Seizure Exhibition on 13-14 March 2014 at the Lumen Gallery in central London and at another showing from 15 May – 8 June 2014 at Swiss Cottage Library Gallery in Camden, London. And it continued at the Beyond Seizures Exhibition at the Institute of Child Health/ Great Ormond Street Hospital Gallery, London, from 28 January-15 July 2015. Wow.

What this was all about and how it happened is a curious tale that started months before at an event funded by the Welcome Trust bringing together epileptics, medical specialists, family members and artists in a unique event arranged by the London Brain Project (LBP), which is a science-art public engagement initiative which provides opportunities for public groups to explore brain sciences through the arts. For me this began on 30 November 2013 when my wife, Gail, and I took part in this unusual workshop where there were a number of tables each led by an artist in a conversation about epilepsy attended by some people with epilepsy, a neurosurgeon and family members.

Each table was to produce an art work from the various views and comments of all concerned and our table was a revelation to me as the group conversation revealed more insight on epilepsy than I had heard in decades of visits to doctors. Using a peg-board our views on various topics were represented by various colours with each contributor using a different colour. In a very short time we had a cavalcade of colour and had not only covered the peg- board but also learnt a lot, our neurosurgeon and others providing some very candid views and insights not out of the medical text books. It was a very interesting and fun exercise but there was more to come.

While talking to our table's artist, Julia Vogl, I showed her a detailed list of all my 72 major fits in the period 1991-2013. Gail had had me document them by severity, location, time of day, duration and possible cause, and this has proved very useful to me in giving explanations to doctors and possibly helping to understand better my type of epilepsy.

But Julia, with her artist's eye, saw this and extracted something much more from this collection of data. She saw how 22 years of my fits could be recorded visually on 72 coloured silkscreen panels stretching a length of 17 metres and one metre high. The specifics of the seizures were represented graphically by different colours and provided an impressive image and definitely a way of seeing epilepsy differently.

Julia's keen artist's eye, along with other contributions from the November workshop, led to the *Beyond Seizure Exhibition* at the Lumen Gallery in March 2014 and the Swiss Cottage Library Gallery in May-June 2014 and at the Great Ormond Street Hospital Gallery in the first half of 2015. The *Timewell Timeline* brought epilepsy into a new colourful light with the large coloured panels bringing a new different energy into the world of seizures.

I have been amazed at what Julia and the *Beyond Seizures Exhibitions* have achieved and the numbers the colourful panels have reached. Getting across a different perception of epilepsy is an important achievement and I am hugely pleased that my 72 fits, with Julia's help, have been able to be seen in a new and enriching context.

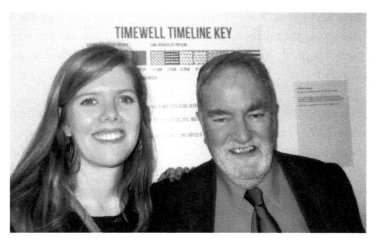

Timewell timeline: Exhibition showing 72 of Steve's seizures turned into art in London. Liberty and Steve in front of Timewell Timeline key.

THE AGE OF RETIREMENT

2009 was an important transition year for the global economy and banking sector and similarly for me too. After 11 years as Editor and five as Editor-in Chief I was now in a new phase in my self- declared title of Editor Emeritus which began when I formally retired in April. I was slowly acclimatising to retirement but that did not mean there was nothing to do at The Banker. The Middle East still needed coverage and at the time I was the best person for it but at a somewhat slower pace.

In this new era of reduced responsibility there were also new opportunities not previously available to a full-time journalist. In early 2009 I had a month or more in Australia visiting family and friends while Gail remained busy at London South Bank University and Liberty was finishing her first year at Cambridge at Homerton College. I was much more of a free spirit now allowing me to really enjoy family pursuits in Australia and traditional Easter pilgrimages to Ardtornish in the Scottish Highlands. But by May I was called to Saudi Arabia and the round of Gulf reports began in earnest.

Nevertheless, the summer allowed us to pursue a long-held ambition to visit Huangshan (or Yellow) Mountain in China for Gail's 60th birthday with old friends Sue Maingay and Chris Tribble. And somehow I managed to chair the *Cross Straits Banking Summit* in Fujian, China for The Banker. In October Liberty's 21st birthday at home provided a joyous occasion for her and 75 pals.

In 2010 I continued to go to Saudi Arabia and elsewhere in the Gulf but after 20 years I handed The Banker's July Top 1000 issue to others and spent a few weeks in Libya, understanding the place and working at the Central Bank of Libya. Little did I know that after a lot of optimism a year later Gaddafi would be dead and Libya in utter chaos. Trips to Nigeria and Washington followed, I had slowed down but there was still fuel in the tank.

December 2010 was important not only for some major events but also because a new book emerged. Our niece, Mari Ericksen, married Shane in Melbourne on the 3rd and not only were we there but also Liberty flew in from China to be bridesmaid. A week later I had my 60th birthday at Chris Ley's house in East Melbourne and I also launched the first book, *Time Well Spent*. And then on the 21st I had another wonderful 60th in London before heading to a holiday in Cairo and Sharm El-Sheikh. A turbulent time but very fortunate for the semi-retired.

2011 was an eventful year which saw the emergence of the Arab Spring, The Banker's 85th anniversary and the Clocks managing extensive travels including Gail and I meeting Liberty in China during her third year of university there. On a reduced schedule I fortunately spent almost a month in Beijing (writing a China diary contained in my 2016 book '*A Decade Well Spent (2004-2014)*', and also visiting Bellagio and Denmark.

I did do some work, a large special report on Nigeria and perhaps my last IMF/World Bank meeting in Washington plus the fifth Top 500 Islamic Banks summit in Malaysia. I was winding down but not finished yet. In December we were joined for Christmas by my sister Margaret and her son Matthew and Dana and their three kids, Caitlin, Frances and Patrick; this included a visit to the ancestors in Devon and then on to Morocco, with Liberty, to visit our friends the Roses in Rabat. My number of seizures had moderated from 10 the previous year to four, again four too many but heading in the right direction.

2012 was another slower transitional year. As usual I thoroughly enjoyed my visit to Saudi Arabia which included playing a little golf with central bank officials. And before the summer Gail joined me in a work trip to Mumbai where I interviewed the deputy governor of the Reserve Bank of India along with the chairmen and CEOs of 15 of India's leading banks for the July issue. Gail took in the museums and the cricket. I also had an extensive visit to China, again meeting old friends, Jiang Jianqing, Chairman of China's biggest bank, ICBC, and Dong Wenbiao, Chairman of China Minsheng Bank, for which I was appointed a consultant.

2012 was London's Olympic year and Gail was extremely active as a volunteer in the press team at the archery events. Another important occasion was Liberty graduating from Cambridge in great style and her starting her career at the UK's Department of International Development (DFID). And in a very curious event I was asked to chair an FT banking conference in Athens entitled '*The Future of Banking in Greece*'.

I survived the event, Greece's banking sector has not done so well since, and we finished the year with a fine Christmas Eve and Christmas Day with friends. I ended the year with four seizures, stable but room for improvement.

2013 was the transition year where play overtook work for both Gail and myself. In the first of a number of big trips we had a wonderful trip through Vietnam which had huge resonance for us, especially in Hanoi, Da Nang and on the Mekong. This delight was preceeded by my cousins' son, David Curtain's curious non- wedding on the beautiful island of Lankawi off Malaysia.

There was work and I filled in for new Middle East Editor, Melissa Hancock, in Kuwait, a very familiar place. Later on I did traditional visits to underbanked India and expanding China but while I was genuinely calming down, my number of seizures was going up.

Doctors, particularly in regard to epilepsy, like to try new approaches and new medications. While changes in pills have caused me grief in the past I agreed with the Queen's Square neurologists to start taking Epilem in mid-March. The new medication caused me problems, however, and I had four seizures, relatively light, in the next two months. This seemed bad, I was not happy and after consultation with my local GP I dropped Epilem and returned to my former medication, Phenytoin. I had seven seizures in 2013, four after moving on to Epilem, and my next seizure was in August, three months after stopping taking Epilem.

Back on my old medication felt better for me and so it remained, the doctors shrugged their shoulders at what Epilem seemed to have done and as I have discovered, at my cost, over the previous 15 years, changing medications has not worked and has had adverse consequences. Is there an answer to this? Can the specialists be blamed? The answer, in my opinion, is no. Reactions to different drugs are different for everybody and, put bluntly, if you don't try you don't know. These are the cruel facts of epilepsy.

Meanwhile, we had planned a big visit to Gail's former stomping ground, Brazil, and this was a fantastic trip covering many parts of Brazil, including the Amazon, and we had a special bonus of being in Rio at the same time as Pope Francis. We are very lucky.

MY SPINAL STROKE
AND ITS AFTERMATH

2014 was a remarkable year not only because of some amazing personal travel in Laos, Cambodia, Australia and Oman along with some traditional work trips to Saudi Arabia and China, but also because of a new dramatic medical experience, a spinal stroke, which occurred in Denmark on 11th July while we were visiting our Danish relatives.

While this narrative is meant to focus on life with epilepsy this year added to my already large and diverse range of medical issues and the stroke was something that had not been foreseen at all. Throughout my life I seem to have amassed a maze of conditions, some self-inflicted, including football injuries, my broken neck (as a result of a seizure) and a certain liking for food which have had their consequences. So before the stroke I was already taking a range of medicines that dealt with epilepsy, type-2 diabetes, blood pressure, high cholesterol and generally being overweight. Known as Tubby Timewell in my youth I did not get any thinner with age. I liked eating and playing golf and while I did use my exercise bike in my study I did nowhere near the amount of exercise I have done in more recent years.

Meanwhile, in July 2014, we were on a short visit to Gilleleje in Denmark for a family occasion and I had felt poorly playing with the children in the garden before lunch. I was fine during lunch but getting up from the table on the back porch I collapsed into the hedge and something was definitely wrong. They got me into the back bedroom but I really couldn't move my legs and my arms were semi-paralysed too. With two nurses present they called for the ambulance. I kept talking, I knew I had to do that and just see what would happen. I kept talking, convincing myself I was still alive and I kept talking in the ambulance, I did not know what was wrong but I felt I was going to talk my way out of it.

In hospital, as often happens, they were not sure what the problem was. I knew that in frontal lobe strokes there was an injection if given within a few hours would do the trick. But doctors were not sure. Both sides, left and right, were not working, I was shunted on to another hospital in Copenhagen for some examinations and then back to the first one at Hillerod. I could at least speak but instead of being paralysed down one side both my legs were affected and my face was fine.

The doctors were in a quandary and the next day after lots of tests and MRIs they figured out I had had a spinal stroke which happens to one in a hundred stroke patients. The chilling aspect of this type of stroke is that while the so-called infarction took place at the top of the spine that is connected to the brain, all the bodily processes going through the spine, such as the bowel and bladder, were affected.

The doctors were in uncharted territory, I was glad I could speak as normal but somewhat like epilepsy and my broken neck in Cairo the outcome was unclear. I was alive but there was a lot of recovery to be done. I could not walk or use my arms but the hospital in Hillerod started working on me and 11 days later I left my Danish hospital (for which I paid nothing) for London. Everything in Denmark went amazingly well and Gail was terrific as always. I was very lucky to have survived all this and to have been given such great treatment by the Danes. Again I was very fortunate.

London was not easy but I had Gail and Liberty by my side. My recovery was in the lap of the gods but I knew it was my willpower that would be the main determinant. Just as with epilepsy and my broken neck I knew with the spinal stroke I had to overcome it and I could not let it get the better of me.

Back home at the end of July we realised we had a holiday booked to Sicily in mid-August. Gail said I could not stand up in the shower, and I couldn't, so how could we go. I was stubborn and took it as a point of principle that I had to go. I could not let this defeat me. I was determined to go and I tried hard with all the equipment and devices available. But I knew the biggest problem was in my attitude and I had to get that right. Despite my poor mobility I convinced Gail we could go and off we went but with considerable trepidation on my part.

With significant help with wheel chairs at airports we made it to a little hotel with its own beach in Syracuse. I had a wheel chair but did not want to use it, I preferred to walk behind it and amazingly I could do it, slowly getting there. Syracuse raised my confidence and my mobility and amongst great weather and great food Sicily had got me going. You have to have goals to overcome in situations like this and success in Sicily provided a great boost to my recovery.

Back in London the real recovery process began with a stroke exercise class at the local gym, the Sobell, and I also began sessions with a private physio in a St John's Wood hospital. Hema, the private physio, got inside my head as well as my body and I quickly saw some improvement. She even convinced me that I could run for a bus. Again, attitude was everything and she made me believe I could run and now I knew I could.

By October people kept saying I had had a remarkable recovery but that was only partially true. I had problems with my bowels and bladder and while Hema had me going up the stairs at home and my mobility had improved considerably, there was still a long way to go and I knew it.

For the rest of 2014 I continued exercise classes, the Physio, swimming and a little running with pilates classes added to the mix, I knew I had to get myself in better shape if I was going to overcome this spinal stroke. December was busy with my birthday, the usual Christmas celebrations with Danish Christmas Eve and Christmas Day itself plus this year we decided to travel to Oman, a delightful traditional Arab country. On New Year's Eve at the new opera house in Muscat we could only reflect on how lucky we were to survive the year in such good form and visit so many good friends in such great places.

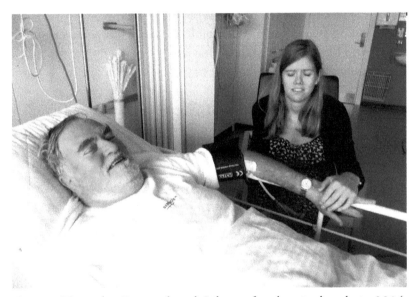

Steve in Hospital in Denmark with Liberty after the spinal stroke in 2014.

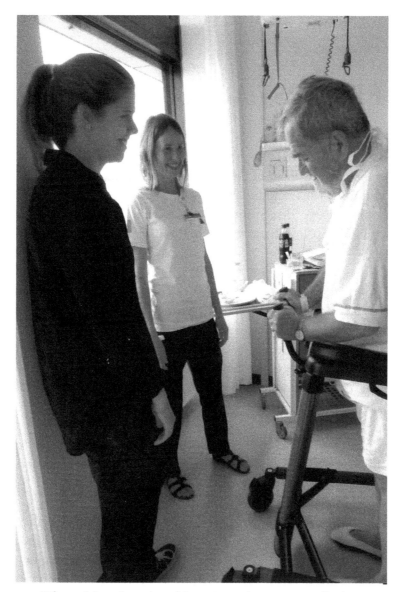

Liberty, Maya (nurse) and Steve in my learning to walk phase.

EPILEPSY ACTION AND ME

Back in the early 1970s I joined the board of the Epilepsy Foundation of Victoria in Melbourne, Australia, as a young person keen to do what I could to help in the wide cause of epilepsy. My enthusiasm has not waned but in my hectic and eclectic life across the globe in the following decades I had not been in a position to contribute greatly to the cause because of work commitments, family and also finding the right vehicle.

In the 2010s in London in semi-retirement I was able to consider more options and look more closely at how I could contribute. One epilepsy conference I attended in London with my wife around 2011 was both interesting and confusing in equal measure. At this first meaningful attempt to get closer to epilepsy I found that there seemed to be many epilepsy charities across the UK, confusion on my part as to what they each did and while there was progress in how epilepsy was dealt with by the medical profession since my first experience in the 1970s, the condition still had the stigmas and prejudices of old and it seemed that not much had changed.

While I noted that my neurologist at Queen's Square in London, JW Sander, was a speaker at this event and the world of epilepsy was obviously changing for the better I did not see what I could do apart from the donations and support.

As it happened at the time I was having a curious combination of seizures and regular nightsweats; although unpleasant all this was neither dangerous nor particularly explainable. As part of the process of analysis and diagnosis a large number of tests, including MRIs etc, were done on me to no great effect. These included an overnight visit to Epilepsy Society's facility at Chalfont St Peter's, near London where various tests were done on my brain.

I was well aware of the pioneering nature of the Chalfont facility over the past hundred years but in all honesty that overnight experience brought forward all the worst fears and thoughts of institutionalisation and I found Chalfont both an unpleasant and unrewarding hospitalisation. I know Chalfont has proved positive for many but that did not happen in my case and rather prejudiced me against the institution.

In time my severe nightsweats eased, possibly because, in my view, of not drinking so much coffee, and this medical issue receded from my radar.

The next pivotal event came a year or two later when Gail and I were invited to attend an epilepsy workshop, arranged by the London Brain Project, a small group funded in part by the Welcome Trust. The London Brain Project is a science-art public engagement initiative which provides opportunities for public groups to explore brain sciences through the arts.

And so Gail and I found ourselves sitting around a table with a neurologist, an artist, other folk with epilepsy and their families trying to produce an art work using a peg-board from the various views and comments of all concerned. As weird as this may sound this format produced for me a more candid discussion of epilepsy, especially from the neurologist, than I had heard in decades of visits to doctors.

The format produced lively and informative discussion, a very colourful art work and an extraordinary aftermath. In this setting I had shown our artist, Julia Vogl, my diary of seizures from 1991- 2013, which I have included an up-to-date version of in the current appendix. She, as an artist, clearly saw something I certainly did not have the imagination to perceive and she amazingly turned my 72 seizures in that period into 72 coloured silkscreen panels stretching a length of 17 metres and one metre high. Her vision is shown in this book as *Timewell's Timeline* and described in the Epilepsy Action article 'How 72 Seizures Became a Work of Art'.

The extraordinary aspect of this is that this Beyond Seizures Exhibition at the Lumen Gallery in London in March 2014 and at two other galleries since bringing a new approach and new vivid colour to the world of seizures and also reaching a new and wider audience. I never thought that my 72 seizures could bring such pleasure and delight to so many.

This positive impact encouraged me to see what I could do further. So I thought I could write some short stories about the positive side of my epilepsy experiences. I gained confidence in the fact that little on a personal basis is written about life with epilepsy and so I contacted Epilepsy Action in Leeds and suggested that I send them a few articles for publication about events in my life.

Epilepsy Action was open and receptive to the suggestion and had a magazine called *Epilepsy Today* which was well suited to this type of personalised article. To my delight they liked and published the articles and those articles, which are included in this book, are in a section called 'The Man with the Memoirs' and are available online also (www.epilepsy.org.uk).

Getting the right tone and getting a positive response was a confidence builder and helped lead me on to doing this book. But while all this was evolving I got to know Epilepsy Action better and I liked their aims to improve the awareness and understanding of epilepsy and to improve the quality and availability of healthcare services for people with epilepsy. And so in getting a better understanding of the charity I learned in 2016 that elections were taking place in that summer to the Board of Trustees.

This seemed a useful thing where I thought I was capable of making, with my business and journalistic background, a good contribution to the welfare of the charity. It was also a new direction for me personally, I had finished my second book in 2016 and I was keen to be useful in something I had had some experience of over my entire life. But I soon realised, once elected, I had a lot to learn still and my first year as a Trustee has been a strong learning experience in picking up on the corporate culture and history of the charity and finding out where and how I can make some contribution.

My first year on the Board of Trustees has been both rewarding and a little frustrating in realising the limitations of what can be achieved. But the structure and finances of the organisation are very sound with a very effective operational management in place. Of course we can all do better but we have an excellent structure in place and I am very pleased to have the opportunity to contribute at the Trustee level to such a solid organisation with a defined purpose and good prospects.

Being on the Board of Trustees has been an eye-opener into the way our charity and other such charities work. We are a team and it is a genuine team effort with a clear objective. This strong ethic gave me confidence that I could add something of a personal nature into this broad mix and hence this collection of memoirs about my personal experience of epilepsy. Building confidence and overcoming adversity are critical issues for those with the condition and I hope these memoirs can be a useful and strengthening experience for readers as they have been for me too.

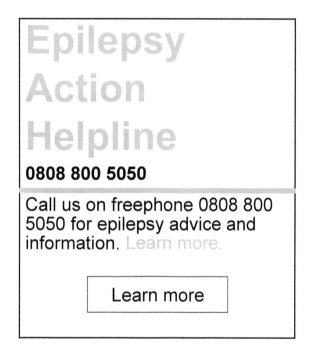

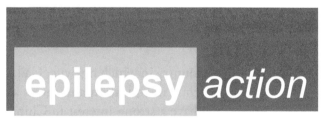

Head Office address
New Anstey House, Gate Way Drive, Yeadon, LEEDS LS19 7XY UK
Phone 0113 210 8800 (UK) or +44 (0)113 210 8800 (international)

EPILEPSY IN CHINA

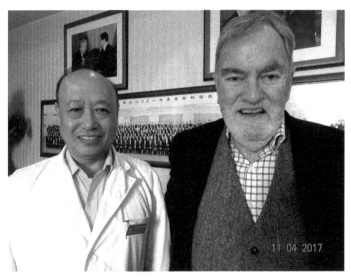

Professor Wenzhi Wang, Chief of the Department of Neuroepidemiology, Beijing Neurological Institute, Beijing Tiantan Hospital with Stephen Timewell in Beijing.

I was fortunate in April 2017 to visit China, a country in which my wife, Gail, and I have worked regularly over the last 30 years or more, she as an academic in education and me as a financial journalist for *The Banker*, part of the Financial Times. We both have a strong interest in China but this visit, unlike many others, was not work, we were visiting our daughter in Beijing who had just been given a three-year posting there with the British government.

In preparations for the visit I mentioned it to Philip Lee, chief executive of Leeds-based Epilepsy Action (British Epilepsy Association) of which I am a recently elected member of the Board of Trustees. Phil was very helpful, as usual, and suggested I try and meet up with Dr Shichuo Li, who is connected to the Beijing-based China Association Against Epilepsy.

Since most epilepsy organisations are primarily national it seemed a huge opportunity to get a better understanding of epilepsy in a country like China which by its sheer size would have more people with epilepsy than any other country.

Dr Li was incredibly helpful and although he was not in China during my visit he recommended and arranged that we see Professor Wenzhi Wang, who is head of the China Association Against Epilepsy, a good colleague of Dr Li, and a professor at the Beijing Neurosurgical Institute at the Beijing Tiantan Hospital, the key focal point for epilepsy in China.

Like all interviews with key officials in China I have learnt from my decades of experience as a financial journalist not to expect too much and while I was fascinated to meet Prof. Wang I had no idea how he would respond.

Everything, however, was in our favour. We had had the proper introductions from Phil Lee and Dr.Li, I was not technically a journalist but a board member of Epilepsy Action in the UK, and to my great delight he was very happy to talk about his organisation, provide figures on epilepsy in China and he understood immediately from the start what I was trying to do, provide a better global understanding of epilepsy.

I could not believe how lucky we were to have made contact with such an open and personable figure and someone who was the key person behind epilepsy in China. You get lucky sometimes and within minutes Prof. Wang had invited us to lunch in two hours time and while we were looking at some relevant medical articles I had another stroke of luck. I accidentally noticed on an article in *The Lancet,* a medical journal, from 2006, the name of one of the writers of this epilepsy piece called JW Sander. I said that Lee Sander was my personal neurologist at Queen's Square in London.

Prof. Wang was amazed by the coincidence and said he knew Prof. Sander well and they had worked together on a large community- based intervention trial in rural China on "The Efficacy Assessment of Phenobarbital in Epilepsy." All this broke the ice and from then on Prof. Wang was even more hugely helpful and encouraging. Having experienced many difficult interviews in Beijing before this was a dream and I was suddenly realising a whole new world of epilepsy was opening up to me.

What was really exciting to discover was not only Prof. Wang's huge enthusiasm for bringing epilepsy treatment to China's rural areas but also the success he was having in the reduction of seizure frequency and the retention of patients on treatment.

The findings in *The Lancet* article of January 2006 showed that the study enrolled 2455 patients and in 68% of patients who completed 12 months' treatment, seizure frequency was decreased by at least 50%, and a third of patients were seizure free. 72% of patients who completed 24 months' treatment had reduction of seizure frequency of at least 50% and a quarter of patients remained seizure free.

The great success of Prof. Wang's "Big Project in Rural Areas" is that since those initial 2006 results the programme has expanded greatly and is cost efficient. The 'Big Project' now covers 100,000 people with epilepsy in 18 out of China's 31 provinces. Prof. Wang acknowledges that today in 2017 the 200 areas now covered only represent about 10% of the population in need, so he says: "There is still a long way to go."

The key, however, is the strategy and the ability to provide treatment relatively cheaply. What seems critical is the approach taken where Prof. Wang focuses on providing just two drugs, phenobarbitone and valproate, old drugs he notes which do not have bad side effects and can be produced cheaply in China. He explains that 100 phenobarbitone tablets, made in China, cost just Rmb1.4 (£0.20) and that each year the central government provides Rmb 17m for the cost of the drugs, not much but enough to make a difference.

This simple approach with these two well-tested drugs provides Prof. Wang with a realistic way forward, more government money would always help but he believes that this strategy is achieving real success, especially in rural areas, where nothing existed before.

For Gail and I we learnt an enormous amount from a standing start in a country which Prof. Wang estimates has 9 million suffering from epilepsy. Given that the World Health Organisation says there are 50 million people worldwide with epilepsy, the China figure could be far higher but as we learned getting accurate figures in large emerging economies such as China can be hugely difficult. Nevertheless, progress on epilepsy in China is definitely being made.

IN HINDSIGHT

Being wise after the event can be relatively easy and allows for a range of options. Being wise before the event is an altogether different exercise which can go horribly wrong. Gauging and analysing events is a critical part of human activity but there is no sure way of providing correct and accurate answers to key questions.

So after over 60 years of having epilepsy are there useful conclusions to be drawn from my experience? In trying to provide some answers it is important to clarify the type of epilepsy one is attempting to describe and a key problem is the huge range of epileptic conditions within what is commonly known as epilepsy.

In my own case, experiencing regular early morning tonic-clonic seizures I have been able to lead a successful career in financial journalism, have a happy family life and, I believe, be a productive member of society. This has not necessarily been the case for many people who have had various forms of epilepsy and have suffered greatly along with their families.

The concept that epilepsy can be extremely diverse and covers a wide spectrum of conditions is not only difficult but makes it extremely problematic for patients to overcome its effects and for them to reach their full potential.

My attempt, in this book, is not to categorise or list the diverse range of epilepsy amongst the over 50 million people worldwide with the condition. The book, in a small way, highlights my experience in overcoming my struggle with epilepsy from child to adult and hopefully gives some examples, in the context of the illness and the problems that emerge from it, of how to cope and how to get on top of its adversities.

My story is not particularly pretty. Bad things have happened over the decades, certainly not as bad as some, but experiences to learn from and build on. It has been a long journey and epilepsy is a journey, which for most people, is something they will never completely understand and something that will never completely disappear. It will be with them all their lives in one shape or form.

The question is not getting rid of it, that is not possible except in a few fortunate cases. The key is learning how to cope, to overcome the difficulties, adapt to the medications with their adverse side effects, and being positive about what can be achieved. The journey is tough, the condition provides its own hurdles and along with them comes the personal challenges.

Attitude can be everything. For patients and their families it is easy to become negative, to accept what the condition brings, to feel sorry for yourselves and follow a downward spiral. It does not have to be that way. Going downhill can be avoided, there can be plenty of positives. Turning negatives into positives is important in creating the right attitude.

I learnt early on as a teenager that I could feel sorry for myself or I could just get on with it. I believe I was lucky enough to take the latter course, helped by strong family structure at home and discipline at school. I was lucky enough to avoid much of the stigma and prejudices attached to epilepsy and I even had the strength of character, somehow, to ignore what my doctors in my teenage years told me I couldn't do.

I was well aware that I could not drive or do related professions but I never accepted I would not finish school or not go to university. I was determined to prove the doctors wrong and I did go to university, even graduate school, and I have had a successful career, becoming Editor of The Banker, part of the Financial Times, in 1992, and I am still Editor Emeritus of The Banker in 2017.

What does all this mean? A cynical type could say my epilepsy was never that bad and I was fortunate enough to lead a relatively normal life with relatively normal successes. That is a possible view but I don't share it.

I agree that my epilepsy has never been as bad as it has been for many people and so I have been lucky. But my early epilepsy, which was debilitating at times, taught me an important lesson, how to cope with adversity. And so in Cairo in 1977 when I had a seizure on a motor bike that I should not have been riding and broke my neck, somehow I had the inner strength to not give up and die as those around me in the hospital did. I carried on, against the odds and with the help of friends, including Gail, my wife, I managed to survive and had the neck re-broken in an Edinburgh hospital two years later.

On the positive side my extremely dangerous Edinburgh operation led curiously to a scholarship to the University of Chicago a year later which has proved to be a core foundation of my career, particularly in London at the Middle East Economic Digest (MEED) and the Financial Times.

Coping with adversity was key for me in the global financial crisis of 2008 where the increased stress of being Editor-in-Chief of The Banker at that time led to more seizures and eventual retirement on ill-health grounds in May 2009. The help from Gail, and daughter, Liberty, allowed me to cope with it all and in 2014 when I had a spinal stroke in Denmark at our relatives I had built up a history of coping with adversity which served me well in those stressful times too.

My life has had more than its fair share of eventful moments. But it is also fair to say that coping with epilepsy has been a critical part of my adventures or journey from childhood to retirement. I have been very lucky in many ways, although some could say I have been unlucky the way events have turned.

But the conclusion to all this, if there is one, and one feels that this cavalcade of stories and tales in this memoir should give some insight, is that the epilepsy condition which I have had for over 60 years has provided both a curious anchor and foundation to my life and in my view has greatly strengthened me and allowed me to cope well with adversity of all kinds. I am grateful for it in many ways and it has clearly helped me develop a positive view of life which I believe has been a real plus in all that I have done. Epilepsy can have its positive side effects too.

Taking a more micro perspective of my six decades with epilepsy what lessons have I learnt about doctors, analysis and different medications? The sheer diversity of form that epilepsy can take is critical in understanding how the medical profession can approach the condition and how patients and their families can deal with it too.

In hindsight doctors are not miracle workers, are not clairvoyant and can, like all of us, make mistakes at times. I fully believe that my consultant Dr Sewell's decision to tell me when I was 14 that I would not finish school or go to university was a bad mistake and many doctors in more recent years have fully agreed.

Analysis of neurological conditions, especially epilepsy, is not an exact science and I fully appreciate the difficulties neurologists and others face. I have learnt throughout my personal experience and more recently as a Trustee of Epilepsy Action that the diversity of the condition varies with almost every patient and there are no strategies that suit all situations.

As I learnt in China in early 2017 from Professor Wang at the China Association Against Epilepsy, some progress has been made in dealing with millions of people in rural areas suffering from epilepsy with a simple combination of uncomplicated, relatively cheap old-fashioned medications. These efforts have helped many to become seizure free but as Professor Wang admits there is still a long way to go. Still a majority of people with epilepsy in the developing world receive no treatment or medication.

The questions raised in China and all around the world are not only how good are the doctors in dealing with the condition but also how good are the medications available now and those being developed? Yes, there are many more medications now than a century ago in Vincent van Gogh's time, for example, but are they effective and do some side effects cause more damage than the original condition?

My personal experience over six decades of taking dilantin (or phenytoin as it is now known) off and on over the period is both mixed and conflicting. My views are not based on a scientific survey but, as can be seen in this book, there have been many periods in my life where I was not on medication or even under medical supervision and it is very hard to gauge whether the medication (mostly phenytoin) when I was taking it made any significant difference to the number of seizures I experienced.

In my 20s and early 30s I had no doctor or medication and had a small number of seizures, around two a year, and this situation continued in my 40s and 50s where I was seizure-free for years at a time even with medication. As the diary of my seizures (contained in the book) shows, my doctors in the last 25 years tried to make me seizure-free with new combinations of drugs at various times but my bad reactions to some of these in the form of severe mood swings and ill affects forced me to abandon these changes and return to my old regulars such as phenytoin.

My wife Gail who has attended me over the last 30 years of intermittent seizures asks whether phenytoin is really effective for me or is it, in effect, just a placebo. I am well aware that different medications react differently on different people and that is a core problem in the diagnosis of epilepsy. Everyone is different. My answer to this vexing question at age 66 is that after dealing with seizures for over 60 years I do not want to try new drugs with new side effects, I do not want mood swings and to upset my family. Being seizure free is an obvious goal but a small number of seizures, for example, one a year, is acceptable if there are no serious, adverse side effects.

While I do not believe that anti-epilepsy medications have worked for me over the past 60 years, I do believe they can work for many people. Finding the right balance, the right medication and the right doctor are all part of the epilepsy puzzle that patients have to cope with and find a solution that works for them. As I said, it is a very inexact science and all those involved from doctors to patients and their families need to have a great capacity to cope with all the obstacles the condition throws up. It is a difficult journey but positive steps can be made.

ACKNOWLEDGEMENTS

'Time Well Spent with Epilepsy' may be a memoir-driven exercise like my two previous books, Time Well Spent and A Decade Well Spent (2004-2014), but it is focussed on a more specific theme, my experience with epilepsy. It is trying to focus on how my epilepsy has affected my life, how it has strengthened me in many ways and how the negative aspects of the condition have been or have become positive drivers in my development.

While this book is different from the others in that it is built around epilepsy, it is hoped that some of the stories involved, viewed in their broader context, can be seen as ways forward for those with the condition. As families play an absolutely critical role in helping those suffering deal with and cope with epilepsy it is important that I acknowledge how magnificent a role my family has played from my childhood years in the 1950s to my current retirement years.

My father, who died in 1975 at the age of 65, was a huge figure in my life and still is, and it was only in my early adult years that I really began to appreciate what he had done to protect and nurture his one and only little boy and his struggle to not allow epilepsy to dim his boy's future.

My mother, Eileen, died in 1956 when I was five, so she did not play a great part in this saga but Dad's next wife, Helena, who entered my life in 1958, was another stabilising and strengthening influence on my life especially in my teenage years when my epilepsy emerged more fully.

In addition I was fortunate to have two older sisters, Margaret (born in 1936) and Julie (born in 1947) who provided strong assistance to me in my early days as well as in more recent years. While in 2017 I was rather shocked to hear from both of them that my first seizures were not when I was 13, as I had thought, but six or so years earlier, I was almost amused when I asked Julie how she had reacted to it all.

She noted, somewhat flippantly: "When we realised that after a long sleep, following a seizure, you were fine again, we stopped worrying."

This was the way it was for me, I had a very caring family, I was lucky, I had problems but I had great support around me and life went on relatively untroubled. For all this I am truly grateful.

While my later teenage years and early 20s proved quite benign my time in Egypt in the late 1970s was quite dramatic from an epilepsy perspective and all through this period and the decades since I was fortunate to have strong stalwart support from my good friend Gail who later became my wife in 1987. She helped steer me through my motor bike seizure in 1977 which broke my neck and nearly killed me. She also attended when my neck was restructured in Edinburgh in 1979 and remained my rock until we finally married in 1987.

Gail has supported me in everything I have done and without her none of what I have achieved would have happened. Also our daughter, Liberty, has been a great source of strength although I regret in the included story '*Telling is Better than Not Telling*' that I had not explained that I had epilepsy and she had to learn about her father's condition the hard way. It was possibly a tough but useful experience in the long run.

Besides family I would also like to acknowledge many friends and work colleagues from across the globe who have been aware of my seizures (I have never hidden it) and have supported me through thick and thin.

I would also like to acknowledge the fine crew at Epilepsy Action and colleagues on the Board of Trustees who have encouraged me to write this book and get across a positive image of epilepsy. Attitude is everything and a positive attitude is key to coping with the condition in all its diverse manifestations.

DIARY OF SEIZURES

The next stage in my epilepsy saga, following my above articles, is the data accumulated about my seizures or fits since the early 1990s. This time frame is beyond the scope of *A Decade Well Spent* but since this data was not included in *Time Well Spent* I thought to include it here as it relates to the extraordinary art exhibition that was built around the data by American artist Julia Vogel that went on to a further exhibition as well.

I enclose the full data collected on my fits since the summer of 1991 and while it is primitive, basic data on the dates and times and details of my seizures over the 24 years, Julia Vogel was able to turn it into a huge, popular art work with pictures 30 metres long (pictures are included). The number of seizures from 2007 to 2014 give some idea of why I was having problems and why I had to retire on ill health grounds in 2009.

In this diary I used the word 'fit' to describe various seizures at the time. The word 'fit' has now been replaced by the word 'seizure' for the condition, but I leave the original wording of the diary as it was when it was written.

STEVE TIMEWELL'S FITS

1991 -   Summer 11am , Elfort Road
1992 -   None
1993 –   None
1994 -   None
1995 -   Summer, early morning Tallin, Estonia

1996 –   18 April, 4.20am at home in Beacon Hill,London 15 November, 7.30am at Beacon Hill

1997 –   None

1998 –   6 April, 7.10am at StokeGabriel, Devon

          6 August, 7am at Les Penots, France

1999 –   15 January, 7.10am at Beacon Hill

          11 February, 6.50am at Beacon Hill

          2 December, 3.30am at Beacon Hill

2000 -   24 March, 6.20am at Beacon Hill

          28 June, 12.30am at Beacon Hill

          13 September, 11.50pm at Beacon Hill

          29 December, 6.40am at Daylesford, Victoria

2001 - ?? March, 9am at Julie's in Melbourne, before Sally's wedding

          13 April, 8am at Ardtornish in Scotland

2002 -   16 February, 8.05am at Beacon Hill

          2 September, 9pm became unconscious at Gwen & Richard's

          2 November, 8pm became unconscious at Eddie's concert

2003 -   None

2004 -   4 January, 7.15am at Beacon Hill

          25 September, 4pm became unconscious at John Lewis

          5 November, 8.30am at Hotel Laleh, Tehran

          12 November, 6am at Beacon Hill

2005 -   7 August, 12am at Beacon Hill just after waking up from return from Cyprus normal fit, standard

          29 September, morning fit on holiday in France with Monash folk, in bed during early morning, sub-standard, a little woozy only

          6 November, evening fit in bed 11pm, flung myself out of bed across the room, probably over tired after China trip

2006 -   1 January, at PJ's in Portsea after exciting New Year's Eve Party where I was probably over tired

2 March, fit in bed early morning (6.30) at Beacon Hill following return the night before from busy schedules in Taiwan and Dubai, again probably over tired plus travel

9 April, fit in bed early morning (7.30) in Ardtornish, Scotland, following motion sickness on drive up to Scotland from London the day before. Also tired and stressed. Stayed in bed most of day

24 May, fit in bed early morning, 5.30am, for 40seconds, busy period during Mike Dowling's visit, probably too much activity

Late July, unconscious after motion sickness twice in ferry trips in Greek islands, dissipated quickly once off ferry

15 August, fit in bed morning, 7.10am, for 40 seconds, no apparent cause, possibly knee injury at the time plus diabetes but not clear- not over-tired

2007 –   5 May, fit in bed at 3am at Beacon Hill, no specific reason, usual tiredness but unexplainable, unusual during the night seizure

16 October, fit in bed at 5.30am, Gail said it was a 'light' fit, I managed to get up and give keynote speech on China at 8.30am, so it was not that bad, clearly I was stressed about the speech and work but nothing unusual in that. Only 2nd fit for 2007.

2008 –   19 January, moderate fit in bed at 7.30am following call from Liberty in Guangzhou, usual aspects, lasted 30 seconds- a minute, slept for a few hours, felt rather bad, no explanation, perhaps stress of press day, perhaps woken by call but it was later on Saturday morning.

17 February Sunday, average fit at 7.30 with long-lasting effects, 45 second, rolled out of bed onto floor, slept for two hours, got back into bed, slept most of day, average, debilitating fit, went to work next day a little worse for wear. Not particularly stressed, press night on the Friday

20 March Thursday, fit in bed at 4.30am in bed at Beacon Hill on Press day before going to Scotland for Easter.

Long fit, stayed in bed, slept for most of day. No reason for fit, no particular stress. 2008 fits maybe related to diabetes.

11 August, Monday, fit in bed at 7am at Beacon Hill before returning to work after three weeks holiday. Average fit, stayed in bed and watched the Olympics. No reason at all for fit, except concern at going back to work.

3 September, Wednesday morning 5.30am on a British Airways flight from Dubai. Four-day working trip with two night flights probably contributed to stress and fit but fit on board was a surprise to me, seemed to be average fit, no major damage done, had to get paramedics to attend at Heathrow and caught taxi home. Slept for Wednesday and stayed home Thursday.

27 September, Saturday morning at 6.30, usual fit , slept most of the day, difficult recovery. Fit followed difficult week in Greece and Awards judging, very busy week, I was concerned on Friday night I had pushed myself hard this week.

29 October, Wednesday morning at 3.10am, usual average fit, woke up and knew something was wrong. Busy at work and a lot to do but no fundamental reason behind this fit, not overly stressed. Stayed in bed and went to naturapath at midday. Feeling fine later in morning but worried by seven fits this year so far.

5 November, Wednesday evening at 9pm after I had gone to bed early. But The night before 2nd Islamic Financial Summit. Normal length fit but recovered soon after, the cause is being worn down by nightsweats and fits, now eight this year. No specific reason except being worn down.

10 December, Wednesday morning at 7am for the usual 50 seconds and slept for the rest of the day. No explanation for this one, night interruptions were light and sweats light, some work concerns but light too – no real reason.

This makes nine this year which is unacceptable.

2009 -   No fits in 2009 due to less stress(retired in April) and more sleep.

2010 –   Friday 29 January at midnight at Julie's house in Melbourne. Relatively short, no particular explanation, no particular cause, could be stress of Aussie visit but unsure of direct cause.

Friday 19 February on flight from Melbourne to Shanghai, about 9 hours into flight. Woke up surrounded by attendants, not sure what happened, bit mouth badly. Managed to fly on to Beijing from Shanghai and then stayed night in Beijing and flew back to London next day. No specific reason for fit, not tired or stressed but had been busy but not enough for fit. Bad to have two fits in two months while away.

Sunday 25 April on flight from London to Riyadh about five hours into flight. Apparently a very mild fit, lasting just a few minutes, I bit my tongue as usual which was more noticeable in the following days. Not very groggy, managed to get off plane unassisted and make it to hotel and have meeting with Oracle and managed to perform well on Monday morning breakfast seminar. Again, no reason for fit, was not worried about event and unclear what prompted fit which was effectively at 3.30 on Sunday afternoon. So three fits in first four months of 2010 and two on planes.

Monday 10 May at 10pm in bed, fell out onto floor. A moderate fit with usual biting of tongue but unexplainable at night after going to bed. No particular stress but in the middle of writing Qatar copy. No real explanation, making four fits in first five months at different times of day. Tuesday 1 June at 6am in bed. A longish fit, usual biting of tongue, stayed in bed all day (Mari and Shane announced engagement). No reason or explanation behind fit, no particular stress. Slept all day and rested the following day. Five fits this year , two on planes, but this one traditional early morning at 6am.

Wednesday 9 June at 12.15 am in bed. A short fit with no significant biting of tongue or damage. I fell out of bed but felt no real ill effects. In the morning. Did not feel great need to sleep all day, a minor fit. But this was the sixth fit this year with two on planes and, at just after midnight, the fits were at different times. No reason behind these latest fits.

Tuesday 15 June at 9.40pm at night soon after going to bed. No real stress and no real tiredness, I had just watched a World Cup match and gone to bed. No explanation for this seventh fit of the year and the fourth in the las five weeks. Bit tongue and mouth feeling troubled.

Tuesday 28 September at 3.15am during the night, a normal length fit but no reason, no stress or particular tiredness. I was sleepy in the morning and stayed in bed. Minor biting of tongue. Eight fits this year.

Sunday 7 November at 10pm after I had gone to bed at 9.30, Gail heard my roar and came up, usual fit lasted a minute, bit my tongue, some blood. I had written the Christmas letter that day and was tired but no real stress or anxiety. Nine fits this year.

Saturday 13 November at 10pm after I had just gone to bed. Gail heard my roar again and came up. Fit lasted a minute and I went off to sleep. No real reason, perhaps concern about the book but no stress. This makes 10 fits this year. Despite a severe social schedule in Australia , the UK and Egypt in December 2010 there were amazingly NO fits, so 2010 total was 10

2011   March 9, at 2.30am in the morning, lasted 50 seconds, made noise and stayed in bed for the rest of the day. No reason for this fit, I had finished the Saudi copy and had had a big meal at Ottolenghi, first fit in almost four months.

June5, at 11pm in the evening on Sunday night in bed, made noise that Gail heard downstairs. I fell out of bed, some blood on sheets. When I woke up got back into bed and slept till Tuesday morning. No reason for this fit, some stress in getting corrections done on Chinese copy but no problem, rested the previous week, no explanation.

October 4 at 12.40am on Monday night after a busy week

2012   February 6, at 1.30pm in the afternoon, a large fit, slept till 4pm fell out of bed and slept for the rest of Sunday and also Monday. This fit was definitely caused by a big two-hour lecture at Cambridge on Saturday 4 Feb. Too much adrenalin and excitement at the lecture but after shopping On Sunday morning I felt terrible and the fit occurred after lunch, I was exhausted and felt it could happen. I had bronchititis as well.

February 14, at 1.30pm in the afternoon. Had spoken to Johanna and then went to bed. Had fit in bed and rolled out of bed onto books, damaged forehead and eyebrow. Stayed asleep for a few hours, no explanation as to why it happened. No reason like the one following the Cambridge Lecture. I stayed in bed that night and the next day too. Not a happy situation and without explanation.

February 28 at 10.20pm in the evening. A normal fit an hour after going to bed, but stayed in bed and slept the next day. Gail heard my yell but I did not do myself any damage. Perhaps this may have been due to the decision to go to Saudi Arabia, who knows? This was the third fit this February, not a good record with no clear explanation.

August 21,2012, at 10.30pm in the evening after going to bed. I rolled out bed and banged my head on the sidetable causing cuts in my face and a lot of blood which Gail cleaned up amazingly. An hour after the fit they put me back into bed and I slept for 36 hours. This was the first fit since February but there was no reason for it or no stress, we were just back from holiday in Bellagio.

2013   March 24, 2013, at 11pm at night in Castle Cottage in Scotland after going to bed at 10pm. Light fit, lasting less than a minute with no loud noises or motion. There was no reason for the fit, we had been walking but no stress at all. I woke up reasonable and we drove to Skye to see the Yeldhams, I did not feel too bad in the morning. I had just started taking Epilem the week before but hard to see any cause. Unusual fit without a cause.

April 20, 2013, around 10am after flight from Hong Kong landing early in the morning, a two-week trip in China. I had gone to bed and must have had fit in bed, bashed my face against the table with some blood, not a bad fit but managed to sleep most of Saturday and Sunday as a result.

May 18,2013, at around 1am in the morning in bed a very light fit which caused no damage and few problems the next day, although I stayed in bed. The fit came on Saturday morning after I arrived back from India on Wednesday, we should have gone to Devon Saturday but I stayed in bed. No real reason for the fit, plenty of rest before it, and nothing to prompt it.

May 29,2013 at 11.53pm in bed. A very light fit that caused no damage. And I slept the next day in bed. There was no reason at all for the fit, I was writing the India copy and I had gone to bed at 9pm. Going to see Dr Battle regarding the Epilem. (Stopped Epilem at end of May after meeting with Dr Battle).

Wednesday 21 August at 9.15pm in bed after going to bed at 8.45. Modest fit in which I stayed in bed, convulsions lasted about a minute, woke up well in the morning with only mouth problems. No reason for this fit but we had been busy with family parties and Liberty going to Melbourne. First fit in three months since I stopped Epilem)

Monday 21 October at 10.30pm in bed shortly after going to sleep. Modest fit in which I stayed in bed . No reason for fit, I had been at Dr Battle's Four hours earlier but was not particularly busy or stressed, I was due to Go to Vienna later in the week. I was very sleepy next day and had meeting at UK Treasury but recovered reasonably well with sleep, again no reason for the fit and no damage done.

Sunday 8 December at 11.40 in bed, only an hour or more after going to sleep following a quiet day. Very mild fit and woke up OK but stayed in bed all day sleeping and went to bed early Monday night. No reason behind this fit but it makes the seventh for 2013 (four due to Epilem)

2014   On Tuesday 25th March at 11.40pm after a very busy day with gold and travel to Saudi being organised I had a short, mild fit in bed lasting about 40 seconds of mild noise and convulsions. I had stopped taking the added Drug the night before. I slept most of Wednesday 26th and only got up on the Thursday, a mild fit, no specific cause except a very busy Tuesday.

On Wednesday 13th August in Ragusa resort of Cavalonga in Sicily at 11.20pm at night not long after going to sleep. Mild fit lasting about 40 seconds in bed and no explanation as to why it should have happened and no reason for the timing late at night. I slept through the following day in the hotel and through the night again, over 32 hours in all and was fine from there.

Friday 29th August at 1.45am in the morning, a very mild fit, not making much noise or doing any damage. Fit was in bed after we had been to see Julius Caesar on the Thursday night. Went to bed at 12. Slept the following day before going out to dinner at Tufnell Park Tavern.

Monday, 15th September, 43 minutes after midnight on the Sunday night. Again a very mild fit, not much noise, came after two late nights, one with Cousin Ian and the other a dinner party with Mark Niall and his wife, Libby. Slept most of the Monday, very quiet, quiet Monday night.

2016   Sunday, 2nd October, at 3am the Cottage Hotel, Devon, on a weekend holiday with sister Margaret and niece Carol. Gail said it lasted the usual 50 seconds, I woke at 4am and slept until 8am. Probably caused by too much excitement at having Margaret over and seeing sister Julie the following day. I recovered remarkably quickly and was relatively unaffected. Two years since my previous fit but annoying since I thought I had got rid of them, not so.

YEAR	No. of Fits
1991	1
1992	0
1993	0
1994	0
1995	1
1996	2
1997	0
1998	2
1999	3
2000	4
2001	2
2002	1
2003	0
2004	3
2005	3
2006	6
2007	2
2008	9
2009	0
2010	10
2011	4
2012	4
2013	7* (4 Epilem)
2014	4 (March,2 August, Sept)

2015	0
2016	1
2017	0 (End of October)
1-1995	2
1996-2000	11
2001-2005	9
2006-2008*	17
2009	0
2010	10 (full year)
2011	4 (full year)
2012	4 (full year)
2013	7* (4 Epilem)
2014	4 (March,2 August, Sept)
2015	0
2016	1

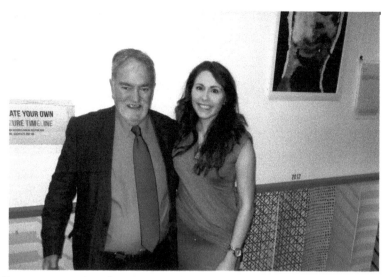

Steve with Michelle Downes, co-founder of the London Brain Project, which arranged the Timewell Timeline.

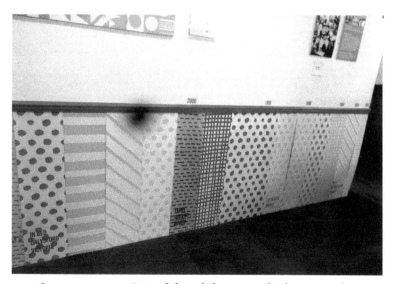

Seizures into art. Part of the exhibition on display in London.

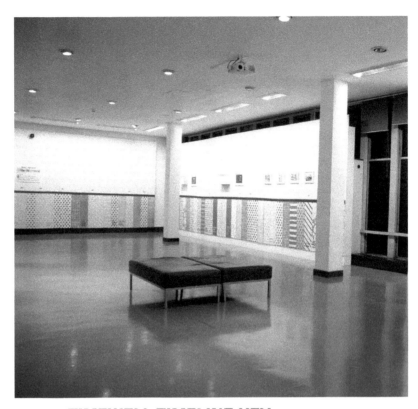

TIMEWELL TIMELINE KEY

SEASON DENOTED BY COLOUR

SPRING SUMMER FALL WINTER

TIME DENOTED BY PATTERN

0-3AM 3-6AM 6-9AM 9-12PM 12-15PM 15-18PM 18-21PM 21-0AM

INTENSITY DENOTED BY BACKGROUND COLOUR

NORMAL SEIZURE

RUGBY TACKLE LIKE, FALL DOWN, HITTING HEAD, BLEEDING OR INJURY TYPE SEIZURE

MOTION SICKNESS INDUCED, GOES UNCONCIOUS SEIZURE

TEXT REFERS TO THE LOCATION OF THE SEIZURE. IF NOT NOTED IT OCCURED @ 29 BEACON HILL IN BED

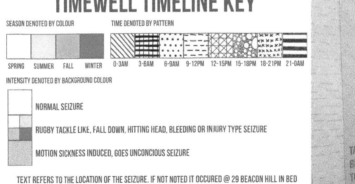

TALIN.
BEFORE FLIGH
TO RIGA

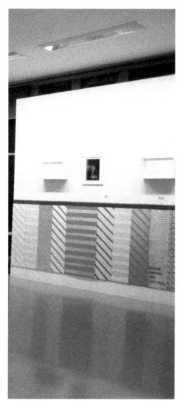

TIMEWELL TIMELINE
Commissioned by London Brain Project
2014
by Julia Vogl
Materials: 17 Meters of hand silkscreened
boards with vinyl and wood.

Description: Working with LBP
on a workshop on Epilepsy, I met
Stephen Timewell who has been ailing
from epilepsy for decades. At the age of
70 he has had 72 seizures. His wife, Gail,
has chronicled them all. I turned her
descriptions and times/dates into a
colourful timeline to express the
situations and seriousness of seizures. There
is a red hand rail that runs the tops of all
the boards, giving them a decorative and
domestic feeling. Many of his seizures
happen as he falls asleeps or wakes.
While he has suffered he has been able
to travel and lead a very successful
and full life despite the disorder.
This work aims to celebrate it.

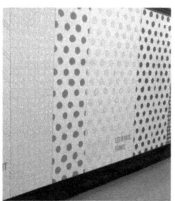

Originally commissioned for
Beyond Seizures show at the Lumen Gallery
the work was shown again at Swiss Cottage
Library Gallery and then again at the
Great Ormand Street Childrens Hospital,
all in London. (between 2014-2015)

More info at:
http://www.londonbrainproject.com/beyond-seizures/

TRAVEL CHART

TIME WELL SPENT WITH EPILEPSY

	2017	2016	2015
JANUARY	MADEIRA*	Devon-Ilfracombe*	OMAN* Liverpool*
FEBRUARY		SOUTH AFRICA	HOLLAND*
MARCH	Devon-Braunton*	SCOTLAND*	
APRIL	CHINA	SCOTLAND*	Wales*
MAY	Chichester*	DENMARK-Bornholm SWEDEN	Birmingham* Wales - Hay*
JUNE		Wales - Hay*	PORTUGAL*
JULY	ITALY, Ancona* Swanage*	GERMANY* AUSTRIA*	Derbyshire* DENMARK*
AUGUST	SCOT,Edinburgh* ITALY, Bellagio* DENMARK, Gilleleje*	GERMANY* FRANCE* Lake District*	DENMARK* SWEDEN* ITALY*
SEPTEMBER		MALTA	ITALY*

OCTOBER	DENMARK	POLAND*
NOVEMBER		
DECEMBER	SPAIN,Madrid* DENMARK	Bradford* Devon*

2014	2013	2012	2011
L A O S * CAMBODIA* AUSTRALIA* AUSTRALIA*	MALAYSIA*VIETNAM*	MOROCCO* US-NY, Redlair*	
			SAUDI ARABIA
	KUWAIT	SAUDI ARABIA	LEBANON
SAUDI ARABIA	CHINA SCOTLAND*	INDIA SCOTLAND*	CHINA
CHINA Hay-on-Wye*	INDIA	INDIA CHINA	CHINA ITALY*
	DENMARK* DEVON*	CHINA	ITALY* SWITZERLAND*
DENMARK*	DENMARK* BRAZIL*	GERMANY* AUSTRIA* DENMARK*	DENMARK*
SICILY*	BRAZIL*	ITALY*	DEVON/ CORNWALL*
		ITALY*	US-Washington,NY

104

DENMARK*   AUSTRIA*   FRANCE -Paris*
                                             DENMARK*
DENMARK*   DUBAI   MALAYSIA
Manchester*
OMAN*   GREECE   DEVON*
                                             MOROCCO*

            CHINA   6*
            SAUDI   11
            ARABIA
            US   9
            DENMARK   8
            ITALY*   12*
            BAHRAIN   3
            DUBAI   4
            QATAR   5
            KUWAIT   4
            GREECE   4

2010	2009	2008	2007
MOROCCO*	CANADA*	AUSTRALIA*	SPAIN*
AUSTRALIA*	US - Chicago*	CHINA ABU DHABI,DUBAI BAHRAIN FRANKFURT	ZAMBIA
AUSTRALIA*	MALAYSIA*		JORDAN
	AUSTRALIA*	SAUDI ARABIA	LEBANON SAUDI ARABIA
SAUDI ARABIA	AUSTRALIA* MALAYSIA* SAUDI ARABIA	BAHRAIN	BAHRAIN
SAUDI ARABIA	QATAR		QATAR
QATAR DUBAI DUBAI			BAHRAIN
	KUWAIT	TURKEY	CHINA-Shanghai
LIBYA	CHINA	DENMARK*	CHINA-Beijing
DENMARK* SARDINIA*	DENMARK* CHINA*	GREECE*	DENMARK* CORSICA*
FRANCE*	LIBYA	ANGOLA	ITALY* UAE
NIGERIA	CHINA FRANCE BAHRAIN		CHINA - Dalian
US-Washington,NY		US-Washington	US - Washington
DENMARK* AUSTRALIA*	DENMARK*		
AUSTRALIA*	JORDAN	US-New York*	CHINA
MALAYSIA* GERMANY* EGYPT*	MOROCCO*	CANADA*	AUSTRALIA*

TIME WELL SPENT WITH EPILEPSY

2006	2005	2004	2003
AUSTRALIA*		DENMARK *	
TAIWAN DUBAI	SAUDI ARABIA PAKISTAN+DUBAI TURKEY	INDIA SAUDI ARABIA	
SWITZERLAND	QATAR	GREECE	
KUWAIT ITALY*			
	KUWAIT	BAHRAIN QATAR	
KUWAIT SPAIN	GREECE SERBIA	S.KOREA UGANDA	
CHINA ROMANIA GREECE*	ICELAND	SPAIN DENMARK CROATIA* GREECE	
DENMARK*	CYPRUS*	GREECE	
SINGAPORE CANADA	US FRANCE* NORTH KOREA CHINA	GREECE* AUSTRALIA US-Washington	CZECH REPUBLIC UAE
		IRAN	IRAN
SPAIN* CHINA	AUSTRALIA*	DENMARK* RUSSIA	TURKEY

Milton Keynes UK
Ingram Content Group UK Ltd.
UKHW050028270824
447345UK00004B/19